T0184652

BestMedDiss

Springer awards „BestMedDiss" to the best graduate theses in medicine which have been completed at renowned universities in Germany, Austria, and Switzerland. The studies received highest marks and were recommended for publication by supervisors. They address current issues from fields of research in medicine. The series addresses practitioners as well as scientists and, in particular, offers guidance for early stage researchers.

Elisabeth Salzer

Identifying Novel Inborn Errors of the Immune System

Primary Immunodeficiencies
with Defective Class Switch
and Autoimmunity

With a Preface by Ass.Prof. Priv.-Doz. Dr. Kaan Boztug

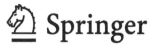 Springer

Dr. Elisabeth Salzer
Vienna, Austria

Dissertation, Medical University of Vienna, 2015

BestMedDiss
ISBN 978-3-658-16795-0   ISBN 978-3-658-16796-7   (eBook)
DOI 10.1007/978-3-658-16796-7

Library of Congress Control Number: 2016961278

Printed on acid-free paper

This Springer imprint is published by Springer Nature
The registered company is Springer Fachmedien Wiesbaden GmbH
The registered company address is: Abraham-Lincoln-Str. 46, 65189 Wiesbaden, Germany

Preface

Rare diseases represent an exceptional challenge to our healthcare system. By definition a single rare disease affects fewer than 1 in 2,000 people. However, as there are up to 8,000 different rare diseases, collectively up to 5% of the European population suffer from a rare disease, often with debilitating and life-threatening consequences. Together with neurologic and metabolic diseases, inborn errors of the immune system represent the majority of rare diseases in humans.

The immune system has to maintain a fine-tuned balance between pro- and anti-inflammatory responses. Apart from pathogen defense it influences a plethora of processes in the human body. Many clinically diverse diseases result from mal-functions of immune surveyor mechanisms. However, these diseases are thought to be of multifactorial origin with both inborn and environmental factors contributing to the pathophysiology. The possibility to define a precise pathomechanism is limited, hindering the discovery of potential novel therapeutic targets. To overcome this problem, model organisms are frequently used and often referred to as potential alternatives with strong caveats with regard to inter-species differences. Therefore, studying patients with rare monogenetic defects of the immune system represent the best possible way to identify critical components and the relevant pathophysiological consequences. Gene discovery in humans used to be tedious and time-consuming and was limited to very large pedigrees and very high disease penetrance. In recent years, high-throughput sequencing technologies have revolutionized biomedical research by allowing insight into the genetic basis of human disease at an unprecedented efficiency. My vision and the focus of my laboratory is that with the advent of state-of-the art genomic technologies, we will for the first time be able to assemble an unbiased and comprehensive view of this complex group of diseases. The recent award of the FWF START Prize and an ERC Starting Grant to myself is testimony to an increasing awareness that rare diseases research at this internationally competitive level can help us understand fundamental biological principles relevant to many human diseases.

The aim of this thesis was to identify critical components of the immune system driving autoimmunity and lymphoproliferation in patients with primary immunodeficiencies. We focused on a cohort of patients with putative autosomal recessive, monogenic diseases and were able to identify 3 novel primary immunodeficiency diseases caused by bi-allelic loss of function mutations in *CD27*, *PRKCD* and *IL21*, respectively.

For CD27 deficiency we described a large cohort of patients with this disease. As all patients shared the same causative missense mutation affecting *CD27*, but displayed diverse clinical presentations, we were able to provide a clinical overview of the disease spectrum. Moreover, we could show that the amount of invariant natural killer cells inversely correlated with Epstein Barr driven lymphoproliferative disease in these patients.

In another patient with severe systemic autoimmunity, we were able to identify a splice site mutation in *PRKCD* encoding protein kinase C delta, which led to complete absence of the protein. The patient displayed glomerulonephritis, was positive for various autoantibodies and previously diagnosed with systemic lupus erythematosus. We could show that in accordance with the previously published role of PRKCD in the literature, this patient exhibited increased mRNA levels of *IL6* after stimulation with Phorbol myristate acetate and showed decreased phosphorylation of the PKCδ target myristoylated alanine-rich C-kinase substrate

(MARCKS). The findings from this study enabled to propose treatment with Tocilizumab, a humanized anti-IL-6 receptor monoclonal antibody currently in use for the treatment of rheumatoid arthritis. PRKCD deficiency is one of the first known, monogenetic causes underlying SLE-like systemic autoimmunity, thus the results of this study are relevant far beyond this individual patient, as they illustrate fundamental mechanisms of disease pathology.

In recent years, we and others have been able to identify monogenetic disease etiologies underlying early-onset inflammatory bowel disease, thereby enlightening our understanding of disease mechanism. In the course of these efforts, we identified IL21 deficiency as a novel cause of early-onset inflammatory bowel disease and immunodeficiency. With the help of *in silico* simulations we demonstrated that the mutated residue is highly conserved and that any change at amino acid position Leu49 would reduce the stability of the native state of the protein. Building on this finding we utilized recombinant wild type and mutated IL-21 protein to demonstrate a loss of function phenotype of the mutant displaying strongly reduced STAT3 phosphorylation upon in vitro cell stimulation. Moreover, as recombinant IL-21 is in clinical trials, we were able to propose an alternative potential curative treatment option for this patient.

Elisabeth Salzer has complete her PhD with distinction in July 2015 and is now specializing in pediatrics and adolescent medicine. Elisabeth shows a strong dedication to the field of immunology and I am sure she will become an excellent physician scientist in the future. She belongs to the very few clinicians who are able to use her background in medicine and combine it with the highest level of molecular research. I congratulate the Springer Best Med Diss selection committee for having selected Elisabeth's thesis for this prize!

Vienna   Ass.Prof. Priv.-Doz. Dr. Kaan Boztug

Acknowledgments

In many perspectives, the time that I could spend in the laboratory at the Center for Molecular Medicine was unique. To be able to interact and work in such a stimulating, creative and motivated environment was and is a privileged situation that I am very grateful for. In professional terms, this was the biggest adventure that I have undertaken so far and there are too many colleagues and friends to be mentioned here explicitly.

Taken together, I would not want to miss the last four years both from a professional and a personal perspective. However, there are people that were simply outstanding in the way they influenced my personal as well as professional development in these last years.

I would like to express my special appreciation and thanks to my supervisor, Kaan Boztug, who has supported me throughout my thesis and has guided me to sharpen and develop my scientific tool set. Over the years I got to know him as one of the hardest-working people I know and I was inspired by his ambitious passion about research and science. He has taught me that persistence and hard work eventually pay off and that knowledge and passion are universal trades that will enable you to do things you never thought you would be able to do.

I would also like to thank my PhD committee consisting of Giulio Superti-Furga and Ulrich Jäger for following my progress and the valuable input and advice I have received from them. Moreover, I would like to express my thanks to Wojtek Garncarz, without whom I could not imagine the last years. His commitment and his high standards have shaped the lab from the beginning and are also a significant factor for its success. I am also happy and grateful that I got to know Ivan Bilic, with whom I had heated scientific discussions and who always made me see the bigger picture.

Together with Elis, Nina, Katharina, Cecilia and Tatjana we mastered crises, burn-outs, weddings, babies, ballroom-dancing, waterfalls, conferences and of course many scientific obstacles we encountered and I am very grateful to know all of you. I would also thank Sola and Stavi who taught me a lot about teaching and supervising and who will both become excellent medical doctors in near future.

Of course I would also like to thank Johannes, my family and friends for their patience in waiting for me to reply to phone calls, show up at dinners and keeping me up-to-date about the really important things in life ☺.

Vienna   Elisabeth Salzer

Declaration

The work of this thesis was accomplished at several academic institutions with the assistance of different collaborators. In the following paragraphs, all contributions are listed in detail.

Chapter 3.1 was published by Salzer, Daschkey et al., 2012. The author of this thesis performed most of the experiments for family A, analyzed and interpreted the data, made the figures and contributed to the manuscript. Sharon Coo, Elisabeth Förster-Waldl, Kirsten Bienemann, Markus G.Seidel, and Arndt Borkhardt cared for the patients, had clinical, therapeutic, and/or diagnostic responsibilities. Elisangela Santos-Valente and Martina Schwendinger helped with exome sequencing and bioinformatic data analyses of family A. Svenja Daschkey, Kirsten Bienemann and Michael Gombert performed exome sequencing and bioinformatic analyses in families B & C. Sharon Choo and Markus G. Seidel arranged and the author of the thesis together with Elisangela Santos-Valente, Sebastian Ginzel, Oskar A. Haas, Gerhard Fritsch, Winfried F. Pickl, Svenja Daschkey and Kirsten Bienemann performed immunophenotypical, functional, and immunogenetic analyses of the patients. Kaan Boztug took overall responsibility for the research performed in this study and wrote substantial parts of the manuscript.

Chapter 3.2 was published by Salzer, Santos-Valente et al., 2013. The author of the thesis and Elisangela Santos-Valente performed most of the experiments, analyzed data and wrote the manuscript together with Kaan Boztug. Stefanie Klaver and Sol A Ban contributed to Western Blot and qPCR analyses. Winfried F. Pickl performed routine immune phenotypic characterization of the patient. Wolfgang Emminger, Andreas Heitger, Klaus Arbeiter, Franz Eitelberger, Markus G. Seidel, Wolfgang Holter, Arnold Pollak and Elisabeth Förster-Waldl provided clinical care and critically reviewed clinical patient data. Leonhard Müllauer and Renate Kain performed histopathological analyses. Kaan Boztug took overall responsibility for the research performed in this study and wrote parts of the manuscript.

Chapter 3.3 was published by Salzer et al., 2014. The author of the thesis performed all experimental work except for B cell class switch and activation assays which were performed by Heiko Sic, Hermann Eibel and Marta Rizzi in Freiburg and T cell proliferation assays which were performed by Winfried F. Pickl. Aydan Kansu, Aydan Ikincioğullari, Esin Figen Dogu, Zarife Kuloğlu, Arzu Meltem Demir and Arzu Ensari provided clinical care of the patient and performed routine clinical interventions. Peter Májek performed computational modeling and *in silico* prediction algorithms. Sol A Ban performed TCR Vβ spectratyping of the patient and Nina Prengemann and Elisangela Santos-Valente assisted in experimental procedures and performed SNP chip based homozygosity mapping. Kaan Boztug conceived this study, provided laboratory resources and together with the author of the thesis planned, designed and interpreted experiments. The author of the thesis and Kaan Boztug wrote the first draft and the revised version of the manuscript.

All chapters of the thesis were written by the author. Kaan Boztug and Ivan Bilic provided critical input to the writing of the thesis.

Reprint permission for all figures in the introduction was obtained from the Nature publishing group through Copyright Clearance Center's Rights Link service.

Table of content

List of Figures

Abstract

Primary immunodeficiencies (Pids) are a complex and heterogeneous group of diseases. In most cases these patients are attributed to a certain PID according to their clinical presentation as a genetic diagnosis can only be established in approximately 40% of the cases. The aim of this thesis was to identify novel monogenic disorders leading to primary immunodeficiencies using state of the art technologies such as exome sequencing and homozygosity mapping. We focused on a cohort of patients with putative autosomal recessive, monogenic forms of PID, presenting with autoimmunity, lymphoproliferation and defective class-switch recombination. In this group of patients we were able to identify 3 novel primary immunodeficiencies caused by biallelic loss of function mutations in *CD27*, *PRKCD* and *IL21*, respectively, leading to 3 publications in peer-reviewed journals.

For *CD27* deficiency we described the largest to-date published cohort of patients with this disease. As all patients shared the same causative missense mutation affecting CD27 (p. Cys53Tyr), but displayed diverse clinical presentations, we were able to provide a clinical overview of the disease spectrum. Moreover, we could show that the amount of invariant natural killer cells inversely correlated with Epstein Barr driven lymphoproliferative disease in these patients.

In another patient we were able to identify a splice site mutation in *PRKCD* encoding protein kinase C delta, which led to complete absence of the protein and resulted in a primary immunodeficiency with severe autoimmunity. The patient displayed glomerulonephritis, was positive for various autoantibodies and was previously diagnosed with systemic lupus erythematosus. We could show that in accordance with the previously published role of *PRKCD* in literature, the patient exhibited increased mRNA levels of *IL6* after stimulation with Phorbol myristate acetate and showed decreased phosphorylation of the PKCδ target myristoylated alanine-rich C-kinase substrate (MARCKS). The findings from this study enabled to propose treatment with Tocilizumab, a humanized anti-IL-6 receptor monoclonal antibody currently in use for the treatment of rheumatoid arthritis.

In a consanguineous family with a history of deaths due to inflammatory bowel disease we identified a missense mutation in *IL21* (p.Leu49Pro) in a boy. With the help of *in silico* simulations we demonstrated that the mutated residue is highly conserved and that any change at amino acid position Leu49 would reduce the stability of the native state. Building on this finding we utilized recombinant wild type and mutated IL-21 protein to demonstrate a loss of function phenotype of the mutant displaying strongly reduced STAT3 phosphorylation upon *in vitro* cell stimulation. Moreover, as recombinant IL-21 is in clinical trials, we were able to propose an alternative potential curative treatment option for this patient.

Taken together the discovery of these three novel PIDs contributed to the understanding of the multifaceted regulatory mechanisms of the immune system and highlighted essential players in these complex signaling networks.

Publications arising from this thesis

Salzer E, Kansu A, Sic H, Majek P, Ikinciogullari A, Dogu FE, Prengemann NK, Santos-Valente E, Pickl WF, Bilic I, Ban SA, Kuloglu, Demir AM, Ensari A, Colinge J, Rizzi M, Eibel H, Boztug K, **Early-onset inflammatory bowel disease and common variable immunodeficiency-like disease caused by IL21 deficiency.** J Allergy Clin Immunol. 2014 Apr 17

Salzer E*, Santos-Valente E*, Klaver S, Ban SA, Emminger W, Prengemann NK, Garncarz W, Müllauer L, Kain R, Boztug H, Heitger A, Arbeiter K, Eitelberger F, Seidel MG, Holter W, Pollak A, Pickl WF, Förster-Waldl E#, Boztug K#.**B-cell deficiency and severe autoimmunity caused by deficiency of protein kinase C δ.** Blood. 2013 Apr 18 (* and # equal contribution)

Salzer E*, Daschkey S*, Choo S, Gombert M, Santos-Valente E, Ginzel S, Schwendinger M, Haas OA, Fritsch G, Pickl WF, Förster-Waldl E, Borkhardt A#, Boztug K#, Bienemann K, Seidel MG#. **Combined immunodeficiency with life-threatening EBV-associated lymphoproliferative disorder in patients lacking functional CD27.** Haematologica. 2013 Mar,13 (* and # equal contribution)

Abbreviations

ADA	adenosine deaminase
AID	activation-induced deaminase
AIRE	Auto-immune regulator
ALPS	Autoimmune lymphoproliferative syndrome
AP3B1	Adaptor-related protein complex 3, beta 1 subunit
APECED	Autoimmune polyendocrine syndrome type 1
APRIL	a proliferation inducing ligand
ATM	Ataxia-telangiectasia mutant
BAFF	B cell activating factor of the TNF family
BCL	B cell lymphoma
BCMA	B cell maturation antigen
BCR	B cell receptor
BLIMP	B lymphocyte induced maturation protein
BLNK	scaffolding protein B-cell linker
BM	Bone marrow
BTK	Bruton's tyrosine kinase
CCR	CC-chemokine receptor
CD	cluster of differentiation
CD40L	CD40 ligand
CGD	Chronic granulomatous disease
CID	Combined immunodeficiency
CVID	Common variable immunodeficiency
CXCL	CXC-motif chemokine receptor ligand
CXCR	CXC-motif chemokine receptor
DCLRE1C	DNA cross-link repair 1C
DN	Double negative
DNA	Deoxyribonucleic acid
DOCK	Dedicator of cytokinesis
DP	Double positive
DZ	Dark zone
EBI2	Epstein-Barr virus induced gene 2
EBV	Epstein-Barr virus
FasL	Fas Ligand
FOXP3	Forkhead box P3
GC	Germinal center
HLA	Human leukocyte antigen
HLH	Hemophagocytic lymphohistiocytosis

aHSCT	allogeneic hematopoietic stem cell transplantation
IFN	Interferon
Ig	Immunoglobulin
IL	Interleukin
iNKT	invariant Natural killer cells
IPEX	Immune dysregulation, polyendocrinopathy, enteropathy and X-linked syndrome
IRF	Interferon regulatory factor
ITK	Interleukin-2 inducible T cell kinase
ITP	Immune thrombocytopenia
JNK	c-Jun N-terminal kinase
LIG	Ligase
LPD	Lymphoproliferative disease
LYST	Lysosomal trafficking regulator
LZ	Light zone
MHC	major histocompatibility complex
MRE11	Meiotic recombination 11-homolog
NBS1	Nijmegen breakage syndrome
NF-κB	nuclear factor kappa-light-chain-enhancer of activated B cells
NHEJ	non-homologous end joining enzymes
NKT	natural killer T cells
PAD	primary antibody deficiency
PI3	Phosphoinoside 3 kinase
PID	Primary immunodeficiency / primäre Immundefekte
PKC	Protein kinase C
PLC	Phospholipase C
PNP	purine nucleoside phosphorylase
PRF1	Perforine 1
RAB27A	Ras-related protein Rab27-A
RAG	Recombination activating genes
RIC	Reduced intensity conditioning
SCID	Severe combined immunodeficiency
SH2D1A	SH2 domain containing 1A
SIN	self-inactivating
SLE	Systemic lupus erythematosus
SNV	Single nucleotide variant
SPENCDI	Spondyloenchondrodysplasia with immune dysregulation
STAT	Signal transducer and activator of transcription
STX11	Syntaxin 11
STXBP2	Syntaxin binding protein 2

TACI	transmembrane activator and CAML interactor
TCR	T cell receptor
TdT	Terminal deoxynucleotidyl transferase
TEC	Thymic epithelial cells
TFH	T follicular helper cells
Th	T helper cells
TNF	Tumor necrosis factor
TNFRSF6	TNF receptor superfamily 6, Fas
Tregs	regulatory T cells
UNC13D	Unc-13 homolog D
UNG	Uracil-N-glycosylase
WAS	Wiskott Aldrich syndrome
XIAP	X-linked inhibitor of apoptosis protein

1 Introduction

1.1 Human Genetics

The understanding of the basic laws of inheritance is essential to study genetic disorders in man. Single gene disorders are rare and often called Mendelian diseases as Gregor Mendel first observed gene segregation patterns by studying selected traits in garden pea *Pisum sativum* (Mendel, 1865). From his work he deduced that basic units of heredity - genes come in pairs, where always one is inherited from each parent. Moreover, he was able to distinguish dominant or recessive traits, by recognizing mathematical patterns in the mode of inheritance.

Mendel's laws of inheritance are stated as follows (adapted from (Mendel, 1865):

1) The Law of Segregation: Each inherited trait is defined by a gene pair. Each gene within a parental pair is called allele. Alleles randomly segregate to the sex cells – gametes so that each gamete contains only one allele of the parental pair. Therefore, during fertilization the resulting offspring inherits one allele from each parent.

2) The Law of Independent Assortment: Genes for different traits are sorted independently from one another so that the inheritance of one trait is not dependent on the inheritance of others.

3) The Law of Dominance: An organism with alternate forms of a gene will express the form that is dominant.

In humans, all genes, except for the X and Y chromosomal ones in males, are present in 2 copies in the cell. Depending on the location of a gene and whether one or two intact copies are needed, a disease phenotype will manifest if a person carries one or two „disease"- alleles. Monogenic disorders can be inherited in four basic modes: autosomal-dominant, autosomal-recessive, X-linked and mitochondrial. Traditionally, monogenic disorders were identified using linkage analyses and candidate gene sequencing. Using this technique loci underlying approximately one-third of Mendelian disorders have been identified (McKusick, 2007). However, in very small, uninformative families, it used to be extremely difficult to identify rare Mendelian diseases due to several reasons such as: incomplete penetrance, locus heterogeneity as well as substantially reduced reproductive fitness (Antonarakis & Beckmann, 2006).

1.2 Exome Sequencing

Before the development of next-generation sequencing technologies, linkage analyses, candidate gene sequencing and positional cloning were the strategies applied to identify disease-causing variants. These strategies mostly focused only on coding areas of the genome while neglecting regulatory regions. However, they have proven to be highly successful in gene discovery. With the development of next-generation DNA sequencing technologies, cost of DNA sequencing decreased dramatically and enabled fast detection of almost all coding variants within a person's genome (Bamshad et al, 2011; Mamanova et al, 2010). Although exome sequencing does not systematically assess non-coding alleles and regulatory regions, it can be applied for the identification of Mendelian disorders, as most disease-causing variants identified until now disrupt the amino acid sequence of proteins (Bamshad et al, 2011).

Today, the major challenge of "gene hunting" using exome sequencing is to distinguish disease-related alleles from the background of non-pathogenic polymorphisms and sequencing errors.

1.2.1   Strategies to identify rare disease causing variants

Exome sequencing of an individual typically yields approximately 20,000 single nucleotide variants (SNVs) out of which more than 95% are known polymorphisms. There are different strategies to identify the disease-causing variant depending on the mode of inheritance, pedigree structure, locus heterogeneity for an investigated trait and inheritance vs. *de novo* emergence of a phenotype (Bamshad et al, 2011). In the past years, since the development of next generation sequencing technologies, causative variants for many Mendelian disorders have been identified. In most of the cases the novel disease-causing variant was identified by filtering against publically available databases, such as dbSNP and the 1000 Genomes project for variants present with a minor allele frequency below 0.01%. This strategy is very powerful especially for rare Mendelian disorders affecting few individuals within a family. In addition, detected SNVs can be further categorized using prediction algorithms, which calculate their potential effect on protein function. Dependent on the mode of inheritance different numbers of cases need to be sequenced in order to identify the disease causing mutation. For recessive disorders in consanguineous families, sequencing of one affected person with the smallest regions of homozygosity should initially be adequate. For non-consanguineous families sequencing of both parents and the affected child is a potent approach to identify potentially disease-causing variants. In any case, optimization of the filtering process tailored to the approach is crucial for the identification of these variants.

1.3   Lymphocyte development

During embryogenesis hematopoietic precursor cells populate the bone marrow (BM). These cells originate from the fetal liver and consist of cells stemming form the aorta-gonad-mesonephros, a part of the mesoderm (Muller et al, 1994) (Pieper et al, 2013)). It is important to consider that hematopoietic stem cells (HCS) do not commit all at once into a certain lineage but as development progresses undergo a certain narrowing towards a specific lineage (Rothenberg, 2000). Long-term reconstituting hematopoietic stem cells (HSC) differentiate into multipotent progenitor cells branching into the lymphoid or the erythro-myeloid lineage (Akashi et al, 2000; Kondo et al, 1997). Due to the expression of *c-KIT* (Waskow et al, 2002) and *FLT3* (Sitnicka et al, 2002) HCSs further mature to common lymphoid progenitors (CLP), thereby loosing long-term self-renewal capacity (Busslinger, 2004). CLPs are a heterogeneous cell population and can give rise to T, B, natural killer (NK) and dendritic cells, depending on the environmental cues. *IL7*, *IL7R* and common γ-chain expression is essential for further differentiation of CLPs (Carvalho et al, 2001; Miller et al, 2002).

The bone marrow provides the appropriate support for the development of B, NK and dendritic cells, while T cells can only develop if a progenitor cell enters a specialized T cell development organ – the thymus.

1.3.1   B cell development

Multiple transcription factors regulate the generation of B lymphocytes from hematopoietic stem cells. The pro-B cell stage represents the earliest stage of committed B cell development (Hardy et al, 1991; Li et al, 1996). Upon induction of *CD19* expression, rearrangement of D and J segments of the heavy chain locus is completed by recombination activating genes (*RAG*) 1 and 2 (Hardy et al, 1991; Li et al, 1996). This stage is followed by a second rearrangement where an upstream V segment is connected to the DJ region (late pro-B cells) (Busslinger, 2004). During this step terminal deoxynucleotidyl transferase (TdT) adds additional nucleotides between the junctions of the rearranged gene segments, which enhances the diversity of the B cell antigen receptor repertoire (Janeway, 2008).

The productively rearranged heavy chain pairs with invariant surrogate light chains (l5 and VpreB) are induced by the transcription factors E2A and EBF. This leads to the formation of a pre-B cell receptor (pre-BCR) on the cell surface (Busslinger, 2004). The productive rearrangement and surface expression of the pre-BCR prevents further heavy chain rearrangement by allelic exclusion, thereby preventing expression of two different BCRs on one cell and leads to proliferation of pre-B cells. Signaling through the pre-BCR requires BLNK and Bruton's tyrosine kinase (BTK) (Janeway, 2008).

After several division rounds large pre-B cells become resting small pre-B cells which re-express *RAG1* and *RAG2* to initiate rearrangement of the immunoglobulin light chain (Meffre et al, 2000). This process is initiated on one allele with joining of V and J segments. Light chains also display isotypic exclusion, so that either the k or l light chain is expressed by one single cell. Productive light chain rearrangement results in the expression of immunoglobulin M (IgM) on the surface of the immature B cell (Meffre et al, 2000). The newly formed B cell receptor complex consisting of IgM and Igα and Igβ is first tested for tolerance to self-antigens in the bone marrow. Cells that react with self-antigens can either undergo apoptosis, clonal deletion, receptor editing, immunological ignorance or anergy. This process is termed central tolerance. Immature B cells with weak reactions to self-antigen are allowed to leave the bone marrow via sinusoids to secondary lymphoid organs to complete development (Janeway, 2008).

1.3.2   T cell development

During embryonic development, the thymus develops from endoderm-derived structures, the third pharyngeal pouch and the third branchial cleft, respectively. It is located above the heart behind the sternum (Hollander et al, 2006). The thymus is populated with hematopoietic cells, thymocytes, intrathymic dendritic cells and macrophages, respectively. It consists of an outer cortex and an inner medulla.

Progenitors enter the thymus at the cortico-medullary junction and move towards the outer cortex (Anderson et al, 1996). Notch ligands expressed on intrathymic epithelial cells guide progenitors to commit them through differentiation (Janeway, 2008; Radtke et al, 1999).

T cell differentiation is defined by surface expression of CD4 and CD8. Initially, progenitors lack most of the surface molecules characteristic for T cells, also CD4 and CD8 and have non-rearranged T cell receptor genes, but express CD3. In the DN1 stage, lymphoid progenitors migrate to the thymus and are predestined to give rise to T cells. However, in this stage they are still not fully committed and are termed "intermediates" (Rothenberg, 2000). It has been shown that these cells can also develop into NK cells as well as dendritic cells (Res et al, 1996). The next commitment towards T lineage occurs with the abrupt induction of members of the Ets and bHLH class A family of transcription factors. In this stage progenitors express the surface markers CD25, CD24 and C-Kit, respectively. The development into NK and DC is strongly attenuated at this stage although still possible. (Rothenberg et al, 1999). There is evidence that TCRαβ and TCRγδ precursors become distinct in this stage before TCR rearrangement (Rothenberg, 2000).

The rearrangement of the T cell receptor β chain starts during the DN2 phase with Dβ to Jβ rearrangement. At this stage T cells start expressing CD25 (Rothenberg, 2002). Subsequently expression of c-Kit and CD44 is reduced, which marks the entry into the DN3 phase. B-selection occurs in this stage as a rearranged β chain is expressed on the surface together with a surrogate α-chain, which enables the assembly of a pre-T cell receptor (pre-TCR), similar to the pre-BCR. With the expression of the pre-TCR, further rearrangement of the β-locus is stopped and, through an intermediate DN4 and immature single positive stage, expression of both CD4 and CD8 on the cell surface is induced, marking the entry in the double positive (DP) phase (Rothenberg, 2002). Large DP cells proliferate and then become small-DP cells, where they only express the TCR at low levels. During this phase positive selection takes place, where the TCR is tested for the ability to bind self-antigens at low level. Positively selected cells, mature and start expressing high levels of the TCR and loose the expression of either the CD4 or the CD8 molecule (Rothenberg, 2002).

1.4 Secondary lymphoid organs and germinal centers

Secondary lymphoid organs contain follicles which, under pathogen free conditions are mainly populated by naive B cells (Victora & Nussenzweig, 2012). Approximately one week after antigen exposure, germinal centers (GCs) develop in these areas and form secondary follicles. During this stage, naive B cells form now the outer border of a GC, the so-called B cell mantle (MacLennan, 1994).

1.4.1 Structure of a germinal center

Germinal centers were first described by Flemming in 1884 as micro anatomical regions of secondary lymphoid organs, that contained dividing cells (Nieuwenhuis & Opstelten, 1984). GCs form a specialized microenvironment within secondary lymphoid organs where B cells undergo proliferation, somatic hypermutation and antigen-affinity driven selection processes (Shlomchik & Weisel, 2012). During this process, BCR affinity plays an essential role in the differentiation step of activated B cells into memory B cells as well as long-lived plasma cells. Anatomically GCs can be separated into dark (DZ) and light zone (LZ). Whereas the dark zone consists mainly of B cells with a high nucleus-to-cytoplasm ratio, LZ B cells are embedded in a network of follicular dendritic cells and T cells (Nieuwenhuis & Opstelten, 1984). These regions are surrounded by a mantle and marginal zone. Phenotypically the cells of the light and dark zone can be distinguished by flow cytometry using markers against the CXC motif chemokine receptor 4 (CXCR4), CD83 and CD86. LZ B cells express CXCR4^{lo}CD38^{hi}CD86^{hi}, whereas DZ B cells are CXCR4^{hi}CD38^{lo}CD86^{lo} (Victora et al, 2010). Tingible body macrophages, which phagocyte dying B cells, are found in almost all GC compartments (Victora & Nussenzweig, 2012).

1.4.2 B cell fate within the germinal center

The dark zone consists of antigen-activated B cells, differentiating into centroblasts while undergoing consecutive rounds of proliferation also termed clonal expansion. During that time somatic hypermutation takes place, enabling higher specificity of the BCR for a certain antigen. Subsequently those centroblasts with best binding to the antigen become centrocytes and migrate further to the light zone of the GC (Klein & Dalla-Favera, 2008). Once B cells engage an antigen via the BCR with sufficient affinity, they up regulate CC-chemokine receptor (CCR)-7 and move to the outer zone of the germinal center, the T cell zone. There activated B cells engage and are stimulated by CXC-chemokine receptor (CXCR)-5 expressing T helper (Th) cells or pre-follicular T helper cells to proliferate further (Fazilleau et al, 2009). Following T cell help, B cells initiate formation of a follicle leading to a GC or initiate extrafollicular plasma cell responses. Until now it is not completely understood which factors determine this differentiation decision (Vinuesa et al, 2009).

During extrafollicular plasma cell responses, B cells up regulate B lymphocyte induced maturation protein (BLIMP)1, maintain expression of the Epstein-Barr virus induced gene (*EBI2, GPR183*) and migrate to junction zones or move to lymph node medullary cords. Here they form clusters of proliferating plasmablasts and by this an extrafollicular response. Some cells undergo isotype switching, but generally these cells are of low affinity and rather short lived. Dependent on the stimulus, extrafollicular responses can last for several weeks and sometimes give rise to somatically mutated autoantibodies (see below) (William et al, 2002). Under normal circumstances, these cells die of an apoptotic death within the secondary lymphoid tissue (Tarlinton et al, 2008).

On the other hand, B cells that up regulate B cell lymphoma (BCL) 6 and reduce EBI2 expression upon interferon-regulatory factor (IRF)-8 expression, differentiate into GC B cells and are targeted to follicles in a CXCR5-dependent manner (Vinuesa et al, 2009). Therefore, most of the B cells in the germinal center display an activated phenotype characterized by the increase in size, polarized morphology and rapid division (Victora & Nussenzweig, 2012). They express high levels of Fas and n-glycolylneuraminic acid as well as high levels of CD38, but loose surface IgD expression. As described above, GC B cells up regulate BCL-6 which is critical for the formation of GCs as mice lacking Bcl-6 cannot form germinal centers and lack high-affinity antibodies (Dent et al, 1997; Ye et al, 1997). BCL-6 also silences the anti-apoptotic molecule BCL-2 maintaining a pro-apoptotic state, which is fundamental in preventing autoimmunity due to defective somatic hypermutation. It also represses p53 and ATR in order to increase the GC B cell tolerance to DNA damage due to AID activity and rapid proliferation (Victora & Nussenzweig, 2012). In addition, BCL-2 reduces expression of Blimp-1, a master regulator of plasma cell differentiation from the GC B cells. It also down-regulates BCR and CD40 signaling, thus guiding B cells towards response to selective signals (Victora & Nussenzweig, 2012).

Since germinal centers are anatomically divided into a dark and a light zone, people sought to decipher whether this also corresponds to functional polarization (Allen et al, 2007). Although light and dark zone cells were similar in complexity and size, gene expression differed in important points. These differences enable to distinguish $CXCR4^{lo}CD83^{hi}CD86^{hi}$ light and $CXCR4^{hi}CD83^{lo}CD86^{lo}$ dark zone cells by flow cytometry.

Marginal zone B cells represent the first line of defense and are capable of mounting a T cell independent response. It has been shown that dedicator of cytokinesis (DOCK) 8 is critical for their development as patients with defective DOCK8 lack marginal zone B cells and do not produce protective antibodies after vaccination (Engelhardt et al, 2009; Randall et al, 2009; Zhang et al, 2009).

Classically cell division is thought to happen in the dark zone whereas cell selection is mainly restricted to the light zone. In line with this hypothesis, it has been shown, that light zone B cells seem to be in an activated state mirrored by the expression of CD69 and CD40, BCR stimulation, as well as nuclear factor (NF)-κB and c-Myc engagement (Victora et al, 2010), whereas mitotic cells can be detected to a higher extent in the dark zone (Hanna, 1964). However, the precise mechanisms guiding cells into one or the other zone remain to be elucidated. This process is illustrated and summarized in Figure 1 taken from Klein & Dalla-Favera, 2008.

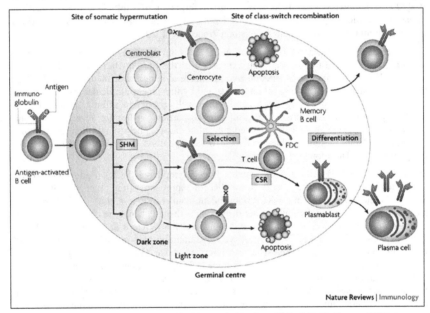

Figure 1:   B cell maturation in the germinal center (taken from Klein & Dalla-Favera, 2008).

1.4.3 Follicular dendritic cells

Follicular dendritic cells (FDCs) reside mainly in the light zone of the germinal center. Their function is to attract germinal center B cells and serve as antigen pool during the germinal center reaction, as they can retain intact antigen on their surface for longer periods of time (Mandel et al, 1981). This trapping of immune complexes on the surface in the form of icosomes mainly relies on complement receptors 1 and 2 (Barrington et al, 2002; Szakal et al, 1985). It has also been shown that follicular dendritic cells secrete CXCR5 and CXCL13/BLC, important chemo attractants for B cells to guide them to the germinal centers (Cyster et al, 2000). In addition, follicular dendritic cells express ICAM-1 and VCAM-1, which are essential for germinal center maintenance and dark and light zone polarization (Haynes et al, 2007). Moreover, the secretion of interleukin (IL)-6 and B cell activating factor of the tumor necrosis factor (TNF) family (BAFF), may be important for a physiologic germinal center reaction (Kopf et al, 1998; Nishikawa et al, 2006; Wu et al, 2009).

1.4.4 T_{FH} cells within the germinal center

Although there are only a small number of T cells within the germinal center, they are critical for affinity maturation of B cells and maintenance of the germinal center. It has been shown that patients with loss-of-function mutations affecting *CD40* or *CD40L* fail to develop germinal centers and exhibit increased levels of non-class switched cells (Allen et al, 1993; Ferrari et al, 2001). Especially the population of T-follicular helper (T_{FH}) cells plays a crucial role within the germinal center. T_{FH} are characterized by the expression of CD4 as well as the B cell zone homing factor CXCR5. On the other hand they down regulate the T cell zone homing factors CCR7 and IL7R. Accordingly, they can be found in B cell follicles and germinal centers, where they interact with antigen-specific B cells in order to facilitate B cell differentiation (Tangye et al, 2013). Upon interaction of naïve CD4 T cells with antigen presenting dendritic cells in the T cell zone, these primed cells up regulate BCL-6 as well as CXCR5 to become early T_{FH} cells. Subsequently, they migrate to the B cell zone where they encounter signal transducer and activator of transcription (STAT) 3 activating cytokines such as IL6, IL12, IL21 and IL27, secreted among others by follicular dendritic cells. This results in up regulation of SAP, MAF, BATF and IRF4, major regulators of the T_{FH} lineage (Tangye et al, 2013). In addition, T and B cell interactions including CD40-CD40L, ICOS-ICOSL and CD28-CD86 are crucial in this developmental phase. It has been shown that not only naive CD4 T cells but also NKT as well as γδT cells can develop into T_{FH} cells in a similar manner (Tangye et al, 2013). Whereas a lot of effort was taken to understand the role of T_{FH} cells in the germinal center, less attention has been paid to CD8 or TH17 cells until now (Victora et al, 2010).

1.5 Inherited disorders of the immune system

Primary immunodeficiencies (PID) are considered a heterogeneous group of inherited diseases that can affect either innate or adaptive immune system separately, as well as their intricate interplay (Al-Herz et al, 2014). Importantly, PIDs have to be distinguished from secondary or acquired immunodeficiencies triggered by pathogens, malignant diseases, immune modulatory treatments or environmental factors (Duraisingham et al, 2014).

Until 3 years ago approximately 200 PID-causing genes have been identified (Al-Herz et al, 2011). In recent years the number increased rapidly. To date, mutations in more than 245 genes have been identified to cause a PID in men (Al-Herz et al, 2014). Nevertheless, even with the identification of a gene defect, the precise pathomechanism of the disease often remains elusive at first but represents a unique opportunity to understand specific aspects of the immune system (Fischer, 2007).

In general, PIDs are under-diagnosed as the primary manifestation can be highly variable but most of the time involves increased susceptibility to infections which can only be evaluated in retrospect (McCusker & Warrington, 2011). However, if unrecognized, the disease can be fatal due to high risk of infections or due to the occurrence of autoimmune phenomena or malignancy.

PIDs are classified according to the primarily affected component of the immune system (Geha, 2007). Defects of the innate immune system include phagocyte disorders, defects in Toll-like receptor mediated signaling and complement disorders. Antibody deficiency syndromes and combined immunodeficiencies (CID) are considered as defects of the adaptive immune system. A unifying clinical presentation is increased susceptibility to recurrent infections and severe infections, or sometimes both, with characteristic susceptibility to certain pathogens, depending on the nature of the immune defect. Moreover, certain forms of PIDs might present with immune dysregulation or even a more complex phenotype where immunodeficiency represents only one of multiple components of the patient's disease (Notarangelo, 2010). The adaptive immune system, comprising the lymphoid compartment, has developed most recently in evolutionary history. Although acting slower than the innate immune response, this system has the ability not only to develop and tailor the highly specific immune answer to foreign, but also to memorize, leading to fast eradication of antigens upon a second encounter. Therefore, in order to understand the development of primary immunodeficiencies, understanding lymphocyte development is crucial. Additionally, the discovery of PID contributed in an essential manner to the understanding of the immune system as we see it today.

1.5.1   (Severe) Combined Immunodeficiencies

Severe combined immunodeficiencies (SCID) represent the most severe forms of T cell immunodeficiencies with an intrinsic impairment of T cell development, sometimes associated with a severe impairment of other hematopoietic lineages.

The disease was first described by Glanzmann and colleagues in 1950 (Glanzmann & Riniker, 1950). SCID results in dramatic susceptibility to pathogens, including especially infections with opportunistic bacteria, viruses and fungi. SCID patients are classified according to the absence or presence of B and NK cells in addition to the T cell defects. As most of the patients succumb to infections within the first year of life, the necessity for a curative treatment is evident. In 1968, the first successful allogeneic bone marrow transplantation was performed in a child with SCID due to a defect in the common γ-chain receptor (Gatti et al, 1968). To date, globally four different molecular mechanisms have been shown to lead to SCID in humans (Fischer et al, 2005). One group includes mutations affecting the common γ-chain of several cytokine receptors. This disease is X-linked and results in absence of mature T and NK cells but presence of CD19+ B cells.

Another mechanism involves increased apoptosis of lymphoid precursors due to defective purine metabolism caused by deficiency of adenosine deaminase (*ADA*), first described in 1972 (Giblett et al, 1972). Later is has been discovered that lymphoid precursors are especially sensitive to the accumulation of deoxyadenosine triphosphate. In addition, it could be shown that the severity of the SCID phenotype corresponds to the residual activity of *ADA* (Hershfield, 2003).

The third group of mutations responsible for a SCID phenotype in humans are defects in pre-TCR/TCR signaling (Liston et al, 2008). For example, somatic rearrangement of both TCR and BCR is essential for lymphocyte differentiation and function. Accordingly, complete loss of function mutations in the recombination-activating genes (*RAG*) *1* and *RAG2* result in SCID with presence of the NK lineage whereas hypomorphic mutations may result in Omenn syndrome (Schwarz et al, 1996; Villa et al, 1998). Taken together, these groups correspond to the majority of SCID patients. Hypomorphic mutations in SCID genes often result in oligoclonal and poorly functioning T cells. Often, the disease is associated with inflammatory and autoimmune manifestations, which can mask the immune defect at first (Felgentreff et al, 2011; van der Burg & Gennery, 2011).

Over the last years an increasing number of this type of diseases have been identified which seem to affect late stages of T cell development. In addition to significant immune dysregulation and severe impairment in pathogen defense, they can also be associated with an increased risk of malignancy. Often, CIDs are furthermore associated with additional B cell defects, either intrinsic or caused by defective T-helper cell activity. Mechanisms of T cell deficiencies are summarized in figure 2 taken from Liston et al, 2008.

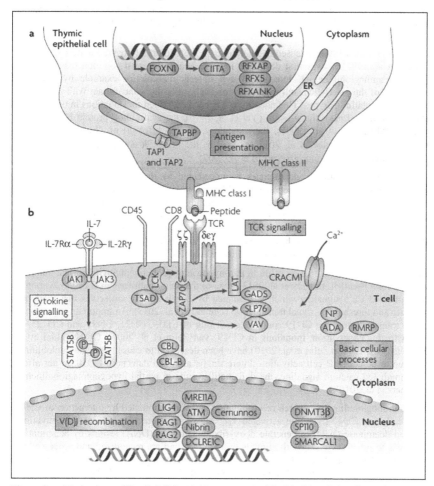

Figure 2: Mechanisms of T cell deficiencies are summarized in this figure (taken from Liston et al, 2008).

1.5.2   Primary antibody deficiencies

Primary antibody deficiencies (PAD) can result from B cell intrinsic defects but also as a secondary effect due to functional impairments in other immune cells such as T or innate immune cells. In general, most of the defective genes highlighted processes involved in B cell development and antibody production (Durandy et al, 2013). However, especially PADs often lack genotype phenotype correlation. This is mirrored by the fact that different mutations in the same gene can lead to distinct phenotypes even with different modes of inheritance (Durandy et al, 2013). Moreover, although most PIDs follow a monogenic pattern of inheritance, some PADs seem to have a more complex genetic basis, also with variable penetrance as exemplified for mutations in the *TNFRS13B* gene (Salzer et al, 2009). Possibly due to this complexity in inheritance and variability in phenotypes the etiology of several PADs is still not known.

The most common PAD is caused by mutations in the Bruton's tyrosine kinase (*BTK*) gene (Vetrie et al, 1993). It was first described in 1952 and is the most common reason for X-linked agammaglobulinemia. Intrinsic B cell defects marked for example by defective expression of the pre-BCR result in absence of mature B cells, concomitant with absence of all immunoglobulin isotypes. This phenotype has been described for mutations in the *l5* chain (Minegishi et al, 1998), the *μ-chain* (Yel et al, 1996), the scaffolding protein B cell linker (*BLNK*) (Minegishi et al, 1999b), the regulatory subunit 1 (p85a) of Phosphoinositide-3-Kinase (*PIK3R1*) (Conley et al, 2012) as well as the *pre-BCR* and *BCR co-receptors Igα* (Minegishi et al, 1999a) and *Igβ* (Ferrari et al, 2007).

Another group of antibody deficiencies is represented by defects in B cell survival and homeostasis which is critically regulated by the two cytokines B cell activating factor (BAFF) and a proliferation inducing ligand (APRIL) (Durandy et al, 2013). Whereas BAFF binds to the BAFF-receptor (BAFFR), the trans membrane activator and CAML interactor (TACI) and the B cell maturation antigen (BCMA), APRIL only bind to TACI and BCMA. Although BAFFR and TACI mutations have been reported to cause PADs in humans many of the described variants can also be found in healthy individuals.

Defects in B cell activation may result in pan-hypogammaglobulinemia with normal numbers of circulating B cells (Durandy et al, 2013). One of the major pathways in B cell activation is BCR-induced Ca^{++} signaling which is regulated by B cell surface molecules that modulate intensity and threshold of signal transduction (Durandy et al, 2013). An important regulator of signal transduction is the CD19 complex consisting of CD19, CD21, CD81 and CD225. In line with this observation, mutations in CD19 (van Zelm et al, 2006), CD21 (Thiel et al, 2012) and CD81 (van Zelm et al, 2010) have been described to cause hypogammaglobuline-mia due to defective B cell activation. Interestingly, although defects in CD20 do not affect BCR mediated calcium signaling, the defect still results in partial hypogammaglobulinemia (Kuijpers et al, 2010).

The immunoglobulin class switch recombination pathway is initiated by interaction of CD40 on B cells and CD40-ligand on activated T_{FH} cells. This interaction induces the activation-induced deaminase (AID) to generate deoxyribonucleid acid (DNA) lesions by deaminating cytosines to uracils. Subsequently, uracils in a DNA strand are recognized and processed by uracil-N-glycosylase (UNG) leading to double strand breaks. Double strand breaks are detected, among others by Ataxia-telangiectasia mutant (ATM) and the MRN complex (MRE11-RAD50-NBS1) and repaired by the non-homologous end joining pathway (NHEJ) leading to class switch recombination. Defects in this pathway usually lead to normal or increased serum IgM levels but reduction or absence of IgG, IgA and IgE. So far mutations affecting CD40 (Ferrari et al, 2001), CD40L (Allen et al, 1993), AID (Revy et al, 2000), and UNG (Imai et al, 2003) have been described. Mutations affecting ATM (Savitsky et al, 1995), MRE11 (Stewart et al, 1999) and NBS1 (Carney et al, 1998; Varon et al, 1998) have also been described but result in syndromes with a broader clinical picture, apart from CSR defects.

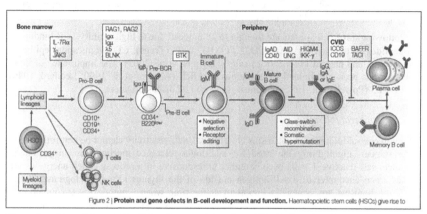

Figure 3:   Gene defects in B cell development (taken from (Cunningham-Rundles & Ponda, 2005)

1.6   Central and peripheral tolerance

Immune tolerance refers to the absence of an immune response to substances or tissues, which are capable of eliciting immune reactions. Dependent on the location of the induction, classifications distinguish central (bone marrow/thymus) from peripheral (lymph node) tolerance. Physiological development of the immune system and the body requires immune tolerance. Whereas central tolerance describes how the immune system learns to distinguish between self and non-self, peripheral tolerance is necessary to prevent over-reactivity of the immune system towards environmental factors such as commensal bacteria or allergens. Even though central tolerance mechanisms work well, not all self-reactive cells can be eliminated as not all self-antigens are expressed in the thymus. Consequently, peripheral tolerance mechanisms are necessary to induce tolerance in these T-lymphocytes (Hogquist et al, 2005).

1.6.1   Central tolerance

Central tolerance is essential for lymphocytes to focus the immune response on pathogens instead of healthy tissue. It takes place either in the bone marrow (B cells) or in the thymus (T cells). During a process called positive selection progenitor T cells able to bind to MHC molecules, are positively selected to differentiate into mature T cells. However, during positive selection self-reactive T cells are also enriched, which increases the risk for autoimmunity. Progenitors with the strongest avidity to self-peptide/MHC complexes are therefore either eliminated during negative selection or made self-tolerant. Thus only weakly reactive progenitors are allowed to mature to take part in immune responses to foreign pathogens (Hogquist et al, 2005).

The process of clonal deletion mainly characterizes central tolerance. This process results in apoptosis of T cells with high affinity for self-antigens (Palmer, 2003). Another process which has mainly been described for B cells is receptor editing. This is a tolerance mechanism where self-antigen binding induces antigen receptor rearrangement either in the T-cell receptor alpha chain or in B cells within the immunoglobulin light chain locus. Another possible tolerance mechanism is anergy, which describes an absent response to antigen even under optimal conditions (Hogquist et al, 2005).

The following three cell subsets are thought to be induced due to high-affinity TCR binding to self-peptides in the thymus: $CD4^+CD25^+FOXP3^+$ cells (Tregs), $CD8\alpha\alpha$ intestinal epithelial lymphocytes and natural killer (NKT) cells (Hogquist et al, 2005). The importance of these processes has been highlighted by mutations in AIRE (Ahonen et al, 1990; Leonard, 1946) and FOXP3 (Powell et al, 1982) in humans (and will be discussed later).

1.6.2 Peripheral tolerance

Although central tolerance mechanisms are efficient, self-reactivity cannot be controlled in all circumstances, highlighting the need for additional tolerance mechanisms. In peripheral tolerance, self-reactive T cells become either unresponsive in a process called anergy or are deleted upon encounter of a self-antigen outside of the thymus (Xing & Hogquist, 2012). These mechanisms are especially important at the time when lymphocytes encounter self-antigens outside of the thymus, such as in the case of developmental antigens, food antigens or antigens only present in times of chronic infection (Xing & Hogquist, 2012).

When T cells encounter a costimulatory signal mediated by CD28 ligation in addition to a TCR signal, they become activated and start to produce cytokines such as IL-2 (Xing & Hogquist, 2012). Activation of the IL-2 receptor complex leads to PI3K/AKT and mTOR mediated T cell proliferation. In case of anergy, mTOR activation is actively suppressed thereby blocking proliferation (Chi, 2012).

1.7 Autoimmunity and auto inflammation

Autoimmunity and auto inflammatory diseases are diseases, which may lead to similar clinical manifestations such as tissue damage and inflammation. However, molecularly they differ in their mechanism. In auto inflammatory disorders the innate immune system directly causes tissue damage for example via altered cytokine production. In autoimmune disorders, the adaptive immune system gets activated and causes tissue damage via autoantibody production or T cell auto reactivity (Doria et al, 2012).

1.7.1 Innate Immune Activation-Auto inflammation

As the innate immune system represents a first line of defense and lacks memory, it relies on the ability of germline encoded receptors to distinguish between foreign and self-antigens (Cheng & Anderson, 2012)). This response is mediated by both complement system and cellular components such as dendritic cells as well as monocytes/macrophages. This response is tightly interconnected with the adaptive immune system and can amplify adaptive immune responses.

To date, syndromes known to result from defects of the adaptive immune system, are for example C1q deficiency, spondyloenchondrodysplasia with immune dysregulation (SPENCDI) and Aicardi-Goutières Syndrome (AGS) (Doria et al, 2012)

1.7.2 Activation of the adaptive immune system - Autoimmunity

B and T cells are unique in their specificity for antigens. Syndromes have been described which highlight the necessity of central and peripheral tolerance mechanisms of the adaptive immune system.

The immune dysregulation, polyendocrinopathy, enteropathy and X-linked (IPEX) syndrome was described in 1982 by Powell (Powell et al, 1982). Clinically, the majority of patients present with watery diarrhea, eczema, diabetes, thyroid autoimmunity, exaggerated response to viral infections and/or an overall increased susceptibility to infections (Moraes-Vasconcelos et al, 2008). Molecularly this syndrome is caused by mutations in the *FOXP3* gene, a key factor for regulatory T cell function. However, also activated T cells transiently express *FOXP3* (Zheng et al, 2010; Zhou et al, 2009). Suppression of immune responses is a complex process and different mechanisms have been proposed (Tang & Bluestone, 2008).

Autoimmune polyendocrine syndrome type 1, also known as APECED is a highly variable disease affecting multiple organs. The diagnosis of APS1 has to include at least two of the three hallmark conditions: autoimmune adrenal insufficiency, autoimmune hypoparathyroidism, and mucocutaneous candidiasis. Descriptions of this syndrome date back to 1910 when the first cases in Finland were described (Ahonen et al, 1990; Leonard, 1946). Most common mutations found in these patients are in the *autoimmune regulator* gene (*AIRE*). This gene is expressed in thymic epithelial cells (TEC) where it regulates expression of self-antigens to be presented to developing thymocytes during positive selection (Derbinski et al, 2005; Derbinski et al, 2001). Recently, some studies have also described *AIRE* expression outside of the thymus in lymph nodes and the spleen (Gardner et al, 2009). It has also been shown that autoantibodies to IL17A and IL17F in these patients are associated with the development of candidiasis (Puel et al, 2010). This is in line with the observation that TH17 responses are essential for fungal immunity (Puel et al, 2011).

Immune dysregulation is also a common feature of some patients with combined immune-deficiencies or patients with leaky-SCID phenotypes (Notarangelo, 2009). For example in patients with *PNP* deficiency, autoimmunity is present in 30% (Notarangelo, 2009). Most commonly patients present with autoimmune hemolytic anemia, however, immune thrombocytopenia (ITP) or neutropenia have been reported as well. It is thought that these complications arise from hyperactive B cells due to loss of T cell regulation (Markert, 1991; Rich et al, 1979). Moreover, patients with *ADA* deficiency or partial DiGeorge anomaly after thymus transplantation can present with autoimmune cytopenias (Notarangelo, 2009). Interestingly, also V(D)J recombination and non-homologous end joining defects can lead to autoimmune cytopenias (Notarangelo, 2009).

Moreover, patients with CVID commonly present with autoimmune manifestations. It has been shown that, depending on country and study, autoimmune manifestations range between 22-48% (Notarangelo, 2009). Also in these patients cytopenias are common and might be the first manifestation of the disease. It has been shown that patients with decreased numbers of regulatory T cells or decreased switched memory B cells together with high $CD19^{hi}$ $CD21^{lo}$ B cells have a higher risk of developing autoimmune cytopenia. However, there is no correlation with organ specific autoimmunity but with splenomegaly (Notarangelo, 2009).

1.8 Lymphoproliferation

In Autoimmune lymphoproliferative syndrome (ALPS) proliferation of double negative T cells (DNT) result from loss of Fas-mediated apoptosis. Canale and Smith first described ALPS in 1967 (Canale & Smith, 1967) as lymphoproliferation simulating malignant lymphoma. However the term ALPS was not used until 1992 when Sneller and colleagues published a „novel lymphoproliferative syndrome resembling murine *lpr/gld* disease" (Sneller et al, 1992). ALPS criteria include persistent lymphadenopathy and/or splenomegaly in the absence of infectious or malignant etiologies, autoantibodies (anti-cardiolipin, anti-nuclear antibodies and a positive direct Coombs test), overt autoimmune disease and the presence of DNT cells. Most commonly these patients present with autoimmune cytopenias (Oliveira et al, 2010). The disease is frequently caused by mutations in the *FAS* gene (*TNFRSF6*) and is inherited in an autosomal dominant way. However, although less frequently, also mutations affecting *FASLG, CASP8, CASP10, NRAS, CTLA4* (ALPS1-5) are known to cause ALPS or a similar phenotype (Al-Herz et al, 2014). The severity depends on the genotype and can vary even among different family members (Jackson et al, 1999). In addition, these patients have an increased risk for developing malignancies of about 10-20% (Straus et al, 2001). Molecularly the disease can be explained by an inappropriate cessation of the immune response (Bidere et al, 2006). Physiologically, a high antigen load can stimulate Fas mediated cell death via up regulation of Fas ligand (FasL) on T cells. In addition, after successful clearance of the antigens, T cells undergo passive apoptosis due to lymphokine withdrawal. In case of defective Fas signaling, activated T cell accumulate and cause autoimmune phenomena.

1.8.1 EBV-driven lymphoproliferation

Epstein-Barr virus (EBV), which was discovered 40 years ago when studying Burkitt's lymphoma, is common in humans and causes infectious mononucleosis in adults. It is a member of the Herpes virus family and persists in the vast majority of people as an asymptomatic infection (Young & Rickinson, 2004). However in patients with underlying immunodeficiencies it may lead to severe immune dysregulation presenting as fatal mono-nucleosis, lymphoproliferative disease (LPD), Hodgkin and Non-Hodgkin lymphoma, lymphomatoid granulomatosis, hemophagocytic lymphohistiocytosis (HLH) as well as dysgammaglobulinemia (Chen, 2011). These manifestations are especially common in patients with defects in important T cell receptor pathway genes, T and B cell interactions or defects in proteins important for the cytotoxic pathway in lymphocytes. Therefore these conditions have been termed hemophagocytic syndromes or familial (primary) HLH (see below). Moreover, a rather heterogeneous group of patients with mutations in *DCLRE1C* (Moshous et al, 2001), *RAG1* and *RAG2* (Schwarz et al, 1996), *SH2D1A* (Coffey et al, 1998), *XIAP* (Rigaud et al, 2006) as well as the *LIG4* (O'Driscoll et al, 2001) gene, can present with lymphoproliferation and immune dysregulation after EBV infection. Within recent years additional immunodeficiencies presenting with lymphoproliferation have been discovered such as *STK4* (Nehme et al, 2012), *MAGT1* (Li et al, 2011) and *ITK* (Huck et al, 2009) deficiency.

1.9 Hemophagocytic lymphohistiocytosis (HLH)

HLH can be a life-threatening clinical condition characterized by extensive and uncontrolled activation of immune cells, especially macrophages. This over activation leads to significant overproduction of IFNγ, IL-6 and IL-10 mirrored clinically by symptoms including splenomegaly, cytopenias, prolonged fever, liver failure, seizures and abnormal NK cell function (Faitelson & Grunebaum, 2014)). Laboratory alterations include elevated soluble CD25, CD168 as well as CD107 surface expression on NK and cytotoxic T cells (Jordan et al, 2011). An important, albeit rare, differential diagnosis includes visceral leishmaniasis, which can present with similar clinical symptoms.

HLH can occur in different clinical contexts and primary (genetic) HLH has to be distinguished from secondary HLH.

Primary HLH is associated with mutations in *PRF1, UNC13D, STX11, STXBP2, RAB27A, AP3B1* (Hermansky-Pudlak type 2) *ATXBP2, SH2D1A (SAP), XIAP, ITK, IL2Rγ, PNP* and *LYST*. Furthermore patients with more complex syndromes such as DiGeorge Syndrome, Wiskott-Aldrich syndrome, chronic mucocutaneous candidiasis, X-linked agammaglobulinemia can present with HLH (Faitelson & Grunebaum, 2014).

In secondary HLH, no family history or genetic cause is evident. It is hypothesized, that HLH is triggered by concurrent infections (EBV) or other medical conditions (malignancy, rheumatologic disorders) (Faitelson & Grunebaum, 2014).

Among triggering infections, EBV infections are most commonly associated with HLH. In this setting the disease course varies between spontaneously resolving and severely life-threatening necessitating HSCT. Among others, especially patients with XLP are at high risk to develop EBV-HLH (Faitelson & Grunebaum, 2014).

1.10 Clinical diagnosis of patients with primary immunodeficiencies

It is well known that PID patients have increased risk for infections, however often non-infectious manifestations such as autoimmunity or auto inflammation may initially be dominant clinical feature. Therefore, PIDs are under-diagnosed as the primary manifestation is highly variable (McCusker & Warrington, 2011). Due to their multifaceted clinical presentations, patients often present to various medical and surgical specialists before the correct diagnosis is made.

Nevertheless, increased susceptibility to infections is the hallmark of the disease. Mostly, patients present with chronic or reoccurring, rarely with unusually severe life threatening infections. Guidelines for diagnosis include infections with opportunistic pathogens, localization/severity of the infection and type of pathogen. In patients with defects in cellular immunity virus and fungal infections are common, whereas patients with antibody deficiencies, are more likely to present with infections with encapsulated bacteria or enteroviruses (Bousfiha et al, 2013). Infections with encapsulated bacteria are also common in patients with complement deficiencies, where they lead to meningitis, bacteremia or septic arthritis. Phagocytic syndromes are often mirrored by infections of skin, lymph nodes, spleen and liver (Lederman, 2000). As specified above, PID patients can also present with signs of autoimmunity/auto inflammation. These clinical manifestations can either be limited to one organ such as thrombocytopenia or autoimmune thyroiditis, or affect several organs.

However, although certain manifestations seem to be autoimmune they rather reflect persistent infections such as enterovirus infection or dermatomyositis (Lederman, 2000). PID may present in a syndromic complex due to additional extra-immune manifestations. Examples are patients with Wiskott-Aldrich syndrome, which exhibit thrombocytopenia, eczema, T and B cell dysfunctions (Aldrich et al, 1954; Wiskott, 1937). This enables clinicians to diagnose the patient prior to onset of immunodeficiency symptoms.

1.11 Therapy of primary immunodeficiencies- curative approaches

1.11.1 Hematopoietic stem cell transplantation (HSCT)

The first successful bone marrow transplantations were performed in 1968 in two SCID patients and one patient with WAS (Bortin, 1970; Gatti et al, 1968). Since then, constant progress has been made to improve transplant-related morbidity and mortality (Filipovich, 2008). High resolution tissue typing, cooperating donor registries and pre- transplant conditioning has led to increased survival of PID patients. Moreover, genetic diagnoses for several PIDs provide additional rationale for transplantation, especially in diseases with natural disease course survival rates below 20 years of age (Filipovich, 2008). For example, severe forms of PID, such as SCID patients, profit from HSCT and this treatment has increased survival rates in these patients to up to 90%.

Dependent on the underlying immunodeficiency, different conditioning regimens have been applied. Albeit HSCT is applied for PID patients since 40 years, there is no clear consensus about donor source or conditioning regimens (Filipovich, 2008). According to the Center for International Blood and Marrow Transplantation (CIBMTR) as well as the European Blood and Marrow Transplant network the type of SCID, predicts early (1–3 years) survival, with better results in T-B+NK- forms and worst outcomes in ADA, specifically with the use of unrelated donors (Myers et al, 2002). A good prognostic factor is young age at transplant (under 1 year, and preferably in the first weeks of life) (Myers et al, 2002).

Myeloablative conditioning regimens often lead to significant transplant-related morbidity and mortality. On the other hand, use of reduced-intensity conditioning (RIC) did not lead to severe acute toxicity in patients with pre-HSCT comorbidities, with the additional advantage of reducing or even avoiding long-term sequelae, especially infertility and growth retardation. On the other hand, RIC are associated with increased probability of mixed donor chimerism and graft rejection. However, mixed donor engraftment is likely to correct for many primary immunodeficiency disorders, but still donor lymphocyte infusion second to HSCT procedures are sometimes required to increase donor chimerism.

Major adverse risk factors are pre-existing co-morbidities and infections prior to HSCT and infections post HSCT. Therefore, early genetic diagnosis maybe even in an asymptomatic state can improve success and the appropriate conditioning regimen can increase the positive outcome of HSCT in PID patients.

1.11.2 Gene therapy

As primary immunodeficiencies constitute a large and heterogeneous group of diseases, gene therapy is only indicated in distinct forms of PID. In addition, in approximately one third of patients no HLA-matched donor can be found. Particularly in those patients gene therapy may represent the best potential curative treatment option (Kildebeck et al, 2012)). In gene therapy the goal is to *ex vivo* correct for/restore gene expression in autologous cells and transplant them back into the patient. Such cells with restored function would revert disease symptoms in the host. To date gene therapy trials have been performed for ADA-SCID (Aiuti et al, 2009; Gaspar et al, 2011b), patients with mutations in the common γ-chain (Gaspar et al, 2011a), patients with WAS (Boztug et al, 2010) and CGD patients (Kang et al, 2011) among others. Whereas gene therapy for ADA-SCID was well tolerated, adverse effects including leukemia were observed with other diseases for reasons still not completely understood (Kildebeck et al, 2012).

In early trials mainly retroviral vectors with strong promoters were used to insert the functional copy into the cells. However as these vectors have a tendency to integrate in the vicinity of gene promoters they can also increase expression of potential oncogenes. Therefore in the last decade, systems were changed to self-inactivating (SIN) lentiviral vectors with endogenous promoters driving transgene expression. In addition these vectors do not depend on active replication of cells for infection and integration (Kildebeck et al, 2012).

Albeit partially successful clinical trials with viral vector systems, transgene silencing due to DNA methylation, insertional oncogenesis and absence of endogenous gene regulation let to efforts to find alternative approaches such as gene targeting using zinc finger nucleases (Porteus & Baltimore, 2003).

Taken together, improvements in the design of viral vectors and the development of new tools for precise gene targeting represent promising strategies for gene therapy trials and might be able to reduce genotoxic side effects.

1.12 Therapy of primary immunodeficiencies- supportive/ non-curative approaches

1.12.1 Enzyme replacement therapy

Unlike other PIDs, in ADA deficiency, another treatment option exists, being enzymatic replacement therapy (ERT) with pegylated bovine ADA (Gaspar et al, 2009). ERT is used as an initial therapy for patients where no related HLA-identical donor is available or where due to risk assessment of the physician ERT was chosen to be the most beneficial treatment option.

1.12.2 Immunoglobulin substitution

Since the 1950s Immunoglobulin (Ig) substitution has been performed for patients with hypogammaglobulinemia. Over the past years the use of Ig has been extended to patients with partial antibody deficiency and patients with combined immunodeficiencies (Group of Pediatric, 2013). This treatment leads to longer life expectancy by reducing infection frequency and lung damage. However, as a human blood product it also bears a risk of infection. It can be administered either subcutaneously or intravenously, with similar efficacy and safety (Group of Pediatric et al, 2013).

1.12.3 Antimicrobials

Although there is limited evidence for prophylactic antibiotics in many PIDs they are widely used. Mostly, common practices are based on knowledge about infecting organisms or studies with patients suffering from acquired immunodeficiencies (Group of Pediatric et al, 2013).

Clear indications for prophylactic antimicrobial therapy are patients with chronic granulomatous disease, since they have a high risk of developing infections with *Staphylococcus aureus*, *Nocardia* and *Burkholderia species*. Patients with humoral immunodeficiencies are at risk of developing bronchiectasis due to chronic lung damage. In this group of patients as well as in patients with hyper-IgE syndrome azithromycin is applied. In T cell immunodeficiencies including SCID patients prophylactic co-trimoxazole is used due to the high risk of *Pneumocystis Jeroveci* infections (Group of Pediatric et al, 2013).

1.12.4 Antifungals

Fungal infections can be challenging to diagnose. However, this type of prophylaxis is mainly limited to patients with CGD, as they show a high risk for developing invasive fungal infections (Group of Pediatric et al, 2013).

2 Aim of the thesis

The aim oft this thesis was to identify novel monogenic disorders leading to primary immunodeficiencies using state of the art technologies such as exome sequencing and homozygosity mapping.

The identification and functional characterization of the underlying genetic defects will help to understand the pathogenesis of these diseases and may open novel therapeutic opportunities for targeted therapy of affected individuals. Moreover, the identification of key-molecules in the development of autoimmunity and/or lymphoproliferation will help to understand the pathophysiology and pathogenesis not only of these monogenic diseases, but can be extrapolated to a large group of diseases involving autoimmunity.

3 Results

3.1 Combined immunodeficiency with life-threatening EBV-associated lymphoproliferative disorder in patients lacking functional CD27

Elisabeth Salzer,[1]* Svenja Daschkey,[2]* Sharon Choo,[3] Michael Gombert,[2] Elisangela Santos-Valente,[1] Sebastian Ginzel,[2] Martina Schwendinger,[1] Oskar A. Haas,[4] Gerhard Fritsch,[5] Winfried F. Pickl,[6][T][SEP]Elisabeth Förster-Waldl,[7] Arndt Borkhardt,[2]#$ Kaan Boztug,[1,7]#$ Kirsten Bienemann,[2]# and Markus G. Seidel[8,9]#$

[1]CeMM Research Center for Molecular Medicine, Austrian Academy of Sciences, Vienna, Austria; [2]Pediatric Oncology, Hematology and Clinical Immunology, Medical Faculty, Heinrich Heine University, Düsseldorf, Germany; [3]Department of Allergy and Immunology, Royal Children's Hospital, Melbourne, Australia; [4]Medgen.at GmbH, Vienna, Austria; [5]Children's Cancer Research Institute, Vienna, Austria; [6]Institute of Immunology, Medical University Vienna, Austria; [7]Department of Pediatrics and Adolescent Medicine, Division of Neonatology, Pediatric Intensive Care and Neuropediatrics, Medical University Vienna, Austria; [8]St. Anna Children's Hospital, Medical University Vienna, Austria; and 9Pediatric Hematology Oncology, Medical University Graz, Austria

(*&# equal contribution)

3.1.1 Abstract

CD27, a tumor necrosis factor receptor family member, interacts with CD70 and influences T-, B-, and NK-cell functions. Disturbance of this axis impairs immunity and memory generation against viruses including EBV, influenza, and others. CD27 is commonly used as marker of memory B cells for the classification of B cell deficiencies including common variable immune deficiency (CVID).

We report the simultaneous confirmation of human CD27 deficiency in three independent families due to a homozygous mutation (p.Cys53Tyr) revealed by whole exome sequencing, leading to disruption of an evolutionarily conserved cystein knot motif of the transmembrane receptor. Phenotypes varied from asymptomatic memory B cell deficiency (n=3) to EBV-associated hemophagocytosis and lymphoproliferative disorder (LPD; n=3) and malignant lymphoma (n=2; +1 after LPD). Two of eight affected individuals died, two others underwent allogeneic hematopoietic stem cell transplantation successfully, a fifth received anti-CD20 (rituximab) therapy repeatedly. Because homozygosity mapping and sequencing did not reveal additional modifying factors, these findings suggest that lack of functional CD27 predisposes towards a CVID-like B cell immunodeficiency and potentially fatal EBV-driven hemophagocytosis, lymphoproliferation, and lymphoma development.

3.1.2 Introduction

CD27 is part of the tumor necrosis factor receptor family and critical for B-, T-, and NK cell function, survival, and differentiation, respectively(1-4). After binding to its specific ligand CD70, CD27 plays a co-stimulatory role highly relevant for antiviral responses, anti-tumor immunity, and alloreactivity(5). CD27 is routinely used as marker for class-switched memory B cells (CD27+IgD- and CD27+IgD+), relevant for the classification of B cell deficiencies including common variable immune deficiency (CVID)(6). Recently, Peperzak et al. showed that CD27 signaling is crucial for sustained survival of CD8+ effector T-cells in mice(7), and Cd27-/- mice show impaired primary and memory CD4+ and CD8+ T-cell responses(4). Thus, it may be hypothesized that constitutional lack of CD27 in humans may cause primary immunodeficiency.

In immunocompetent hosts, primary Epstein Barr Virus (EBV) infection is often asymptomatic, whereas in immunodeficiencies such as IL-2-inducible T-cell kinase (ITK) deficiency, X-linked lymphoproliferative syndromes (XLP1, XLP2), familial hemophagocytic lymphohistiocytosis (HLH) and others, EBV infection may lead to persistent symptomatic viremia(8-11). Although EBV-specific immunity involves virus-specific humoral components, CD8+ effector T-cells are considered essential for long-term virus control(12). Here, we report on eight pediatric patients originating from three independent pedigrees, who lack functional CD27 and presented with EBV-associated lymphoproliferative disorder (EBV-LPD, n=3) with or without HLH, with malignant lymphoma (n=2, +1 after LPD) or were clinically asymptomatic (n=3).

3.1.3   Methods

Patients: Material from patients and healthy donors was obtained upon informed consent in accordance with the Declaration of Helsinki. Family-A was analyzed in Vienna, Austria, while families-B and -C were assessed in Düsseldorf, Germany. The study was approved by the respective institutional review boards.

Flow cytometric analysis: Analysis of CD27 surface expression and B cell class switch was performed as described earlier(13).

DNA isolation and Primer Design: See Supplementary Appendix.

Homozygosity mapping: Genome-wide genotyping based on Affymetrix® Genome-Wide Human-SNP-Array-6.0 was performed for all five family members of family-A. For homozygosity mapping, DNA of each core family member was diluted to 50ng/µl in 12µl. The protocol was carried out according to the manufacturer's instructions. Raw data were analyzed using genotyping console version 4.0.1.8.6. Loss of heterozygosity (LOH) analysis was performed as well as genotyping, followed by more detailed analysis using PLINK. Homozygous regions in all family members were detected using PLINK, using a window size of 5000bp with a minimum of 50 SNPs within this region(14). Adjacent intervals were considered to represent a single interval when the distance between the adjacent intervals was <1MB in size. Based on these data, homozygous regions present exclusively in the most severe affected patient as well as homozygous regions present in all three affected siblings were detected (Supplementary Tables 1 and 2).

Exome sequencing and data analysis: Exome sequencing for family A was performed in Vienna, while families B and C were assessed in Düsseldorf, Germany. For family A, a 50 base pair paired read multiplexed whole exome sequencing (WES) run was performed for the most severe affected patient on a Illumina HiSeq2000 Sequencer running on HiSeq Control Software (HCS) 1.4.8, Real Time Analysis Software (RTA) 1.12.4.2. For WES, DNA was diluted to 20ng/µl in 57µl and sample preparation was carried out using Illumina TruSeq DNA Sample Preparation Guide and the Illumina TruSeq Exome Enrichment Guide. The multiplexed pool of six samples including the patient was run on eight lanes. Demultiplexing and raw image data conversion was performed using Consensus Assessment of Sequence and Variation version 1.7. (CASAVA). Reads were aligned using BWA using the algorithm for short reads (up to ~200bp)(15), a gapped global alignment with maximum of 1bp gap open to a human genome 19 (hg19) reference was performed. Insertion/ deletion realignment and GATK base quality score recalibration was performed(3). Single nucleotide variants (SNVs) and Insertions/Deletions were called using Unified Genotyper and GATK Variant quality score recalibration (1000Genomes, hapmap, dbSNP131) was performed. All thresholds for GATK tools were based on the GATK Best Practice Variant Detection v3 recommendations. SNV and insertion/deletion lists were uploaded to SeattleSeq Annotation database. Variants present in 1000Genomes and dbSNP were excluded and lists were filtered for nonsense, missense and splice-site variants within the homozygous regions detected in the most severely affected patient. For families B and C, a similar approach was taken with minor differences referring to the usage of single reads with 100 cycles and alignment with BWA for long reads and usage of dbSNP132 dataset. Resulting variation calls were annotated by NGS-SNP(16) using a local copy of the ENSEMBL databases, PolyPhen2(17), SIFT(18) and ConDel(19) before imported into an SQL database.

3.1.4 Results

Patient Reports and Immunological Findings. Patient one (family-A, Figure 1A), a five-year old girl from a Turkish consanguineous family presented at the age of 17 months after severe primary infectious mononucleosis with suspected hemophagocytic lymphohistiocytosis (HLH); a brief summary of her clinical phenotype was described as correspondence recently(20). She developed fulminant EBV-LPD and systemic inflammatory response syndrome, and was treated repeatedly with high-dose steroids and rituximab over four years. Flow cytometry revealed undetectable CD27+ lymphocytes (Figure 1B), an increase of transitional and CD21low B cells, and near-absent invariant natural killer T (iNKT) cells (Tab. 1; and Supplemental Figure 2). Two of her siblings, patients two and three (Figure 1A), were clinically asymptomatic but showed borderline hypogamma¬globulinemia (Tab.1, and Supplementary Appendix).

Patient four (family-B, Figure 1A) presented at 18 months of age with EBV-LPD and HLH, and was treated according to the HLH-2004 protocol (including dexamethasone, etoposide, cyclosporine-A) plus rituximab. Nine months after initial presentation, EBV-LPD relapsed without signs of hemophagocytosis. He again received HLH treatment and rituximab, followed by matched unrelated cord blood transplantation. The younger sister of patient four, patient five (Figure 1A), is 16 months old. She was diagnosed with absent CD27 expression and EBV-infection only after the CD27 defect had been identified in her brother.

Patient six (family-C, Figure 1A) presented at the age of 15 years with EBV-LPD. He responded to rituximab, but EBV-viremia recurred three months later. Although he was hypergammaglobulinemic at diagnosis and his peripheral B cells returned four months after rituximab, immunoglobulin levels slowly decreased. Approximately 20 months after initial presentation, a relapse of EBV-LPD occurred, progressing into T-cell lymphoma within four months and requiring treatment with rituximab and chemotherapy (R-CHOP, see Supplementary Appendix) followed by matched unrelated cord blood transplantation. Flow cytometric analysis at relapse revealed absent CD27+ lymphocytes and iNKT cells (Tab.1). From the patient's two older sisters, patients 7 and 8, only limited clinical history and no immunological data were available. Both died of suspected EBV-driven T-cell lymphoma at 2 and 22 years of age, respectively (Figure 1A), and the diagnosis of CD27 deficiency was established retrospectively from Guthrie card DNA (see below).

Genetics. Because of the variability of phenotypes in family-A, we performed homozygosity mapping and whole-exome sequencing (WES) after earlier detection of the CD27 mutation by conventional Sanger sequencing (Wolf et al., manuscript in preparation), to exclude other underlying disease-causing or –contributing genetic conditions and to define whether the mutation in CD27 alone was sufficient for the development of a phenotype. Single-nucleotide-polymorphism (SNP)-array based homozygosity mapping in family-A revealed four intervals which were present only in the affected sibling (patient 1; Supplementary Table 1). However, WES did not reveal any additional relevant genetic aberrations (Figure 1C). Analyses of all three individuals lacking CD27+ cells (patients 1-3) revealed a total of two overlapping, homozygous candidate intervals (Supplementary Table 2), including an interval on Chromosome 12 containing the CD27 gene. The missense mutation in CD27 (c.G158A, p.Cys53Tyr) was found homozygous in three of four siblings in this family and heterozygous in both parents (Figure 1D).

The notion of parental consanguinity and shared ethnic background (Lebanese) in families-B and -C suggested a common autosomal recessive genetic alteration. Therefore, WES of patients four and six was performed which identified the same missense mutation (c.G158A) in CD27 as the only novel shared homozygous single nucleotide variant predicted to be deleterious or probably damaging by different prediction tools (Supplementary Results and Supplementary Figure 1 and 3). The mutation was confirmed by Sanger Sequencing in all cases (Figure 1D). It is located within a motif of the ligand-binding domain evolutionarily conserved among different species and various TNFR family members (Supplementary Figure 4). Retrospective analysis of patients 7 and 8, who had died years earlier, using DNA obtained from Guthrie newborn screening cards confirmed the same CD27 mutation (Supplementary Figure 1); unfortunately, no specimens for immunological analyses were available from those patients.

3.1.5   Discussion

Presented clinical and laboratory observations revealed a novel CD27-linked immuno-deficiency predisposing towards an EBV-associated, potentially fatal, disease. In parallel, van Montfrans et al. recently identified a different homozygous mutation in CD27 (c.G24A, p.Trp8X) in two brothers of a consanguineous Moroccan family, of whom one died from severe infectious mononucleosis at young age and the other recovered with persistent EBV-viremia and secondary hypogamma¬globulinemia(21). The clinical courses of patients 1-8 and the patients reported by vanMontfrans et al. suggest that the immunologic/environmental context of the primary EBV infection might play a role for the first occurrence of hypogammaglobulinemia and the severity of the clinical symptoms in CD27-deficient patients(21), although longitudinal observation of a larger number of patients, and, ideally, preemptive monitoring of asymptomatic family members, will be needed to confirm this hypothesis. While „Timing and Tuning" was described necessary for costimulatory signals by Nolte et al.(5), and other TNF- or immunoglobulin receptors (e.g. herpes virus entry mediator [HVEM], CD30, OX40 [CD134], 4-1BB [CD137]or CD28) have partially overlapping functions (reviewed in (22)), the present human data suggest that CD27 might not be essential but unique among costimulatory molecules in its relevance for the primary immune response against EBV. Together, the identification of CD27 deficiency in four independent families and the observation that no additional mutations in genes other than CD27 could be identified by WES suggest that CD27 deficiency alone, either due to a complete lack (p.Trp8X) or deficient surface expression (p.Cys53Tyr), is disease-causing with broad clinical variability.

Immunologic Consequences. The absence of iNKT cells in CD27-deficient patients during massive EBV-LPD (i.e., patient 1 and 6; Table 1, Supplemental Figure 2) may indicate a primary role of iNKT cells for EBV-LPD pathogenesis as described in SAP, XIAP, and ITK deficiency(9, 23, 24), implicating that the CD70-CD27 axis acts as a co-stimulatory requirement for iNKT cells, or it may be a secondary phenomenon.

Other clinically relevant consequences of CD27 dysfunction might include i) decreased memory formation to viral (including vaccine protein) antigens(4, 25), and ii) perturbed anti-tumor immunity of T cells(26), γδT cells(27), and NK cells(28, 29), potentially leading to an increased risk of other malignomas in addition to EBV-lymphomas.

It is likely that more individuals with dysfunctional CD27 will be identified among patient cohorts with hypogammaglobulinemia (±EBV-LPD) and absent CD27-expressing memory B cells, potentially leading to the recognition of CD27 deficiency as a novel, albeit probably very rare, CVID-like memory B cell deficiency(30-32). Of note, patients one and three also showed expansion of transitional and CD21low B cells, which is reportedly associated with increased risks of lymphadenopathy, splenomegaly, and granuloma formation in CVID, similar to XLP patients(33).

Conclusions. CD27 deficiency should be considered in all patients with hypogammaglobulin-emia or unusually severe causes of EBV infection in order to allow for an individualized treatment based upon the hitherto existing experience with this condition. Our results illustrate that modern genomic technologies such as WES may identify and confirm disease-causing mutations in monogenetic recessive diseases even with limited numbers of affected persons. Future studies to elucidate the cellular pathomechanistic consequences of CD27 deficiency are warranted.

3.1.6 Acknowledgements

The authors thank the patient families and the staff of the immunology outpatient clinics and hematology-oncology wards for their cooperation, Drs. H. Gadner, E. Förster-Waldl, A. Heitger, and G. Mann (Vienna) for their support of experimental analyses, clinical advice, and insightful comments, and Dr. S. Ehl and his team (Freiburg) for critical review of the manuscript and HLH diagnostics including NK cell assays. Authors from Vienna thank Drs. M. Eibl and H. Wolf for referral of family-A and constructive discussions. Funding of parts of this work was provided by the Deutsche Forschungs¬gemeinschaft (to KBi).

3.1.7 Authorship

MGS, KBi, AB, and KBo prepared the manuscript; SC, KBi, MGS, and AB cared for the patients or had clinical, therapeutic, or diagnostic responsibilities; ES, EVS, MS and KBo performed homozygosity mapping, whole exome sequencing and bioinformatics analyses in family A; SD, KBi, and MG performed exome sequencing and bioinformatic analyses in families B and C; ESV, SG, OAH, GF, WFP performed immunophenotypical, functional, and immunogenetic analyses; MGS and KBi prepared the table; SC edited the manuscript.

3.1.8 Disclosures

No author has any financial or other potential conflict of interest to disclose.

3.1.9 References

1. Bigler RD, Bushkin Y, Chiorazzi N. S152 (CD27). A modulating disulfide-linked T cell activation antigen. J Immunol. 1988 Jul 1;141(1):21-8.

2. Camerini D, Walz G, Loenen WA, Borst J, Seed B. The T cell activation antigen CD27 is a member of the nerve growth factor/tumor necrosis factor receptor gene family. J Immunol. 1991 Nov 1;147(9):3165-9.

3. Gravestein LA, Amsen D, Boes M, Calvo CR, Kruisbeek AM, Borst J. The TNF receptor family member CD27 signals to Jun N-terminal kinase via Traf-2. Eur J Immunol. 1998 Jul;28(7):2208-16.

4. Hendriks J, Gravestein LA, Tesselaar K, van Lier RA, Schumacher TN, Borst J. CD27 is required for generation and long-term maintenance of T cell immunity. Nat Immunol. 2000 Nov;1(5):433-40.

5. Nolte MA, van Olffen RW, van Gisbergen KP, van Lier RA. Timing and tuning of CD27-CD70 interactions: the impact of signal strength in setting the balance between adaptive responses and immunopathology. Immunol Rev. 2009 May;229(1):216-31.

6. Klein U, Rajewsky K, Kuppers R. Human immunoglobulin (Ig)M+IgD+ peripheral blood B cells expressing the CD27 cell surface antigen carry somatically mutated variable region genes: CD27 as a general marker for somatically mutated (memory) B cells. J Exp Med. 1998 Nov 2;188(9):1679-89.

7. Peperzak V, Xiao Y, Veraar EA, Borst J. CD27 sustains survival of CTLs in virus-infected nonlymphoid tissue in mice by inducing autocrine IL-2 production. J Clin Invest. 2010 Jan 4;120(1):168-78.

8. Dupre L, Andolfi G, Tangye SG, Clementi R, Locatelli F, Arico M, et al. SAP controls the cytolytic activity of CD8+ T cells against EBV-infected cells. Blood. 2005 Jun 1;105(11):4383-9.

9. Huck K, Feyen O, Niehues T, Ruschendorf F, Hubner N, Laws HJ, et al. Girls homozygous for an IL-2-inducible T cell kinase mutation that leads to protein deficiency develop fatal EBV-associated lymphoproliferation. J Clin Invest. 2009 May;119(5):1350-8.

10. Williams H, Crawford DH. Epstein-Barr virus: the impact of scientific advances on clinical practice. Blood. 2006 Feb 1;107(3):862-9.

11. Filipovich AH. Hemophagocytic lymphohistiocytosis and other hemophagocytic disorders. Immunol Allergy Clin North Am. 2008 May;28(2):293-313, viii.

12. Moosmann A, Bigalke I, Tischer J, Schirrmann L, Kasten J, Tippmer S, et al. Effective and long-term control of EBV PTLD after transfer of peptide-selected T cells. Blood. 2010 Apr 8;115(14):2960-70.

13. Kuzmina Z, Greinix HT, Weigl R, Kormoczi U, Rottal A, Frantal S, et al. Significant differences in B-cell subpopulations characterize patients with chronic graft-versus-host disease-associated dysgammaglobulinemia. Blood. 2011 Feb 17;117(7):2265-74.

14. Purcell S, Neale B, Todd-Brown K, Thomas L, Ferreira MA, Bender D, et al. PLINK: a tool set for whole-genome association and population-based linkage analyses. Am J Hum Genet. 2007 Sep;81(3):559-75.

15. Li H, Durbin R. Fast and accurate long-read alignment with Burrows-Wheeler transform. Bioinformatics. 2010 Mar 1;26(5):589-95.

16. Grant JR, Arantes AS, Liao X, Stothard P. In-depth annotation of SNPs arising from resequencing projects using NGS-SNP. Bioinformatics. 2011 August 15, 2011;27(16):2300-1.

17. Adzhubei IA, Schmidt S, Peshkin L, Ramensky VE, Gerasimova A, Bork P, et al. A method and server for predicting damaging missense mutations. Nat Methods. 2010 Apr;7(4):248-9.

18.	Kumar P, Henikoff S, Ng PC. Predicting the effects of coding non-synonymous variants on protein function using the SIFT algorithm. Nat Protoc. 2009;4(7):1073-81.

19.	Gonzalez-Perez A, Lopez-Bigas N. Improving the assessment of the outcome of nonsynonymous SNVs with a consensus deleteriousness score, Condel. Am J Hum Genet. 2011 Apr 8;88(4):440-9.

20.	Seidel MG. CD27: A new player in the field of common variable immunodeficiency and EBV-associated lymphoproliferative disorder? J Allergy Clin Immunol. 2012 Feb 24.

21.	van Montfrans JM, Hoepelman AI, Otto S, van Gijn M, van de Corput L, de Weger RA, et al. CD27 deficiency is associated with combined immunodeficiency and persistent symptomatic EBV viremia. J Allergy Clin Immunol. 2011 Dec 24.

22.	Croft M. Costimulation of T cells by OX40, 4-1BB, and CD27. Cytokine Growth Factor Rev. 2003 Jun-Aug;14(3-4):265-73.

23.	Pasquier B, Yin L, Fondaneche MC, Relouzat F, Bloch-Queyrat C, Lambert N, et al. Defective NKT cell development in mice and humans lacking the adapter SAP, the X-linked lymphoproliferative syndrome gene product. J Exp Med. 2005 Mar 7;201(5):695-701.

24.	Rigaud S, Fondaneche MC, Lambert N, Pasquier B, Mateo V, Soulas P, et al. XIAP deficiency in humans causes an X-linked lymphoproliferative syndrome. Nature. 2006 Nov 2;444(7115):110-4.

25.	Xiao Y, Peperzak V, Keller AM, Borst J. CD27 instructs CD4+ T cells to provide help for the memory CD8+ T cell response after protein immunization. J Immunol. 2008 Jul 15;181(2):1071-82.

26.	Song DG, Ye Q, Poussin M, Harms GM, Figini M, Powell DJ, Jr. CD27 costimulation augments the survival and antitumor activity of redirected human T cells in vivo. Blood. 2012 Jan 19;119(3):696-706.

27.	DeBarros A, Chaves-Ferreira M, d'Orey F, Ribot JC, Silva-Santos B. CD70-CD27 interactions provide survival and proliferative signals that regulate T cell receptor-driven activation of human gammadelta peripheral blood lymphocytes. Eur J Immunol. Jan;41(1):195-201.

28.	De Colvenaer V, Taveirne S, Delforche M, De Smedt M, Vandekerckhove B, Taghon T, et al. CD27-deficient mice show normal NK-cell differentiation but impaired function upon stimulation. Immunol Cell Biol. Oct;89(7):803-11.

29.	Sugita K, Robertson MJ, Torimoto Y, Ritz J, Schlossman SF, Morimoto C. Participation of the CD27 antigen in the regulation of IL-2-activated human natural killer cells. J Immunol. 1992 Aug 15;149(4):1199-203.

30.	Chapel H, Lucas M, Lee M, Bjorkander J, Webster D, Grimbacher B, et al. Common variable immunodeficiency disorders: division into distinct clinical phenotypes. Blood. 2008 Jul 15;112(2):277-86.

31.	Alachkar H, Taubenheim N, Haeney MR, Durandy A, Arkwright PD. Memory switched B cell percentage and not serum immunoglobulin concentration is associated with clinical complications in children and adults with specific antibody deficiency and common variable immunodeficiency. Clin Immunol. 2006 Sep;120(3):310-8.

32.	Cunningham-Rundles C. Common variable immunodeficiency. Curr Allergy Asthma Rep. 2001 Sep;1(5):421-9.

33.	Wehr C, Kivioja T, Schmitt C, Ferry B, Witte T, Eren E, et al. The EUROclass trial: defining subgroups in common variable immunodeficiency. Blood. 2008 Jan 1;111(1):77-85.

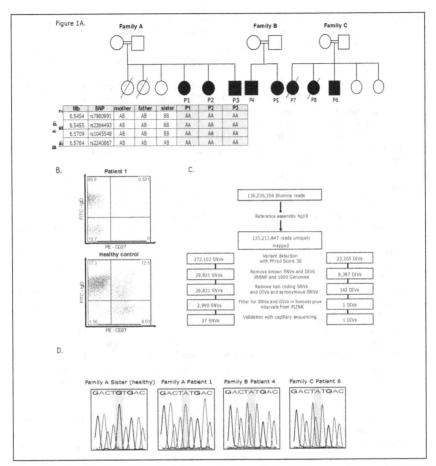

Figure 4: Identification of CD27 deficiency in three kindreds. Three pedigrees with CD27 deficiency were identified. Family A was analyzed by homozygosity mapping, revealing a homozygous interval on Chromosome 12 (A). Two siblings of patient 1 (Family A) had died at 9 months and three days of age, respectively, of unknown causes without molecular diagnosis in Turkey; no material for immunologic or genetic analyses was available (A). Flow cytometry showed absent surface expression for CD27 in lymphoid cells including B cell subsets, shown here in patient 1 for IgD vs. CD27 staining on CD19-gated B lymphocytes (B). Next generation sequencing was performed in patient 1 for homozygous intervals detected exclusively in patient 1 (C). None of the total of 28 additional variants were validated using capillary sequencing, suggesting that the mutation in CD27 is causative of the phenotype in patient 1 (C). Sanger sequencing confirmed the same mutation in CD27 (c. G158A, p. Cys53Tyr) in patients 1-3 from family A, patient 4 and 5 from family B, and patient 6-8 from family C, respectively (D). The CD27 mutation shows perfect segregation in family A, including heterozygosity in the parents and a homozygous healthy state in the unaffected sister (D).

Table 1: Patient characteristics and immune phenotypical details of CD27 deficient individuals.

Patient	1	2	3	4	5	6
Centre	Vienna	Vienna	Vienna	Melbourne	Melbourne	Melbourne
Gender	Female	Female	Male	Male	Female	Male
Ethnic origin	Turkish	Turkish	Turkish	Lebanese	Lebanese	Lebanese
Current age	5 years	14 years	3.5 years	4 years	16 months	19 years
Age at onset	15 months	NA	NA	1 year	1 year	15 years
Symptoms	Recurrent EBV-LPD, SIRS	None, asymptomatic	None, asymptomatic	EBV-LPD, EBV-HLH	Fever, EBV+ ulcers	EBV-LPD, recurrent sinusitis, lymphoma
Treatment	IG; Steroids; Rituximab*	None	IG† from age 4-20 months	HLH-2004, cord-HSCT	None	Rituximab, R-CHOP, cord-HSCT
IgG before treatment, g/L (reference range)	4.51 (4.45-15)	8.43 (6.98-11.9)	2.9 (0.55-7.99)	4.67 (2.86-16.8)	11.6 (2.86-16.8)	32.4 (5.18-17.8)
IgA before treatment, g/L (reference range)	0.55 (0.21-2.03)	0.67 (0.22-2.74)	0.09 (0-0.64)	1.1 (0.19-1.75)	1.2 (0.19-1.75)	3.93 (0.33-2.67)
IgM before treatment, g/L (reference range)	0.581 (0.36-2.28)	1.34 (0.19-0.99)	0.56 (0.09-0.77)	0.75 (0.43-1.63)	0.85 (0.43-1.63)	0.85 (0.32-1.35)
EBV plasma load, copies/ mL min-max	1e2-2e6¶	ND	0-3.6e2§	0-5e6¶	8e6	0-5e6¶
EBNA Ab	NA (IVIG)	Positive	Positive	ND	ND	ND
Response to vaccination antigens	Tetanus low Pneumococcus not vaccinated HiB low TBE low-normal	Tetanus normal Pneumococcus normal HiB normal TBE normal	Tetanus low-normal Pneumococcus low-normal HiB low TBE normal	Tetanus normal Pneumococcus ND HiB normal	Tetanus low-normal Pneumococcus ND HiB normal	Tetanus normal Pneumococcus no response** HiB normal
CD19+ B cells, number/µL	490-1100	520	750-1040	1120	1700	84
IgD-CD27+ B cells	Absent	Absent	Absent	Absent	Absent	Absent
transitional B cells, % CD19+	↑ 47	ND	↑ 24	ND	ND	2.6
CD21low B cells, % CD19+	↑ 38	ND	↑ 18	ND	ND	0.4
CD4+ T cells, number/µL	1340	1540	1460	1660	2400	796
CD8+ T cells, number/µL	2150	1210	1280	1250	1580	2724
NK cells, number/µL	320	260	310	270	250	293
iNKT cells, % of CD3+	<0.01%-0.02%	0.08%	0.09%	ND	0.02	<0.01%
in vitro T cell proliferation*	Normal	ND	ND	Normal	ND	Normal
NK cell function†	Mildly reduced	ND	ND	Moderately reduced	Mildly reduced	Mildly reduced
EBV-specific T cells‡	Present, with increased IFNγ secretion	ND	ND	ND	ND	ND

Table legend: NA, not applicable; EBV-LPD, EBV-associated lymphoproliferative disorder; SIRS, systemic inflammatory response syndrome; EBV-HLH, EBV-associated hemophagocytic lymphohistiocytosis; IG immunoglobulin replacement; CyA, cyclosporin A; cord-HSCT, allogeneic cord blood hematopoietic stem cell transplantation; R-CHOP, rituximab / cyclophosphamide/ doxorubicin/vincristine/ prednisolone; ND, not determined; reference range, age-specific ranges of immunoglobulin levels in parenthesis; Pneumococcus, pneumococcal polysaccharide vaccine; HiB,

Haemophilus influenzae B vaccine; TBE, tick-borne encephalitis vaccine; IFNg interferon-gamma; [*]
in vitro T cell proliferation was measured as standard lymphocyte function test after three day
incubation with phytohemagglutinin (in patients 1, 4 & 6), and concanavalin A, pokeweed mitogen,
CD3, Tetanus antigen, and staphylococcal superantigens (patient 1); [+]NK cell function: cytotoxicity
assay with peripheral blood mononuclear cells against NK-sensitive target cells (K562) in six different
effector and NK:target-cell ratios; [‡] cytokine secretion assay, EBV peptivator; [§] two courses of
rituximab in one year; [||]stopped 2 years ago; [¶]always pos. when B cells present, [#]variable,
asymptomatic, [**] performed when patient became hypogammaglobulinemic.

3.2 B-cell deficiency and severe autoimmunity caused by deficiency of protein kinase C d

Elisabeth Salzer,[1] Elisangela Santos-Valente,[1] Stefanie Klaver,[1,2] Sol A. Ban,[1] Wolfgang
Emminger,[3†]Nina Kathrin Prengemann,[1] Wojciech Garncarz,[1] Leonhard Mu̇llauer,[4] Renate Kain,[4]
Heidrun Boztug,[5] Andreas Heitger,[5] Klaus Arbeiter,[3] Franz Eitelberger,[6] Markus G. Seidel,[5] Wolfgang
Holter,[5] Arnold Pollak,[3] Winfried F. Pickl,[7†]Elisabeth Förster-Waldl,[3] and Kaan Boztug[1,3]

[1]CeMM Research Center for Molecular Medicine of the Austrian Academy of Sciences, Vienna,
Austria; [2]Instituto de Ciencias Biomedicas, Universidade de Sao Paulo, Sao Paulo, Brazil;
[3]Department of Pediatrics and Adolescent Medicine, [4]Clinical Institute of Pathology, and [5]Department
of Pediatrics, St. Anna Kinderspital and Children's Cancer Research Institute, Medical University of
Vienna, Vienna, Austria; [6]Department of Pediatrics and Adolescent Medicine, Klinikum Wels-
Grieskirchen Wels, Austria; and [7]Christian Doppler Laboratory for Immunomodulation and Institute
of Immunology, Center for Pathophysiology, Infectiology and Immunology, Medical University of
Vienna, Vienna, Austria

(*equal contribution)

3.2.1 Abstract

Primary B cell disorders comprise a heterogeneous group of inherited immunodeficiencies,
often associated with autoimmunity causing significant morbidity. The underlying genetic
etiology remains elusive in the majority of patients.

In this study, we investigated a patient from a consanguineous family, suffering from
recurrent infections and severe lupus-like autoimmunity. Immunophenotyping revealed
progressive decrease of CD19[+] B cells, defective class switch indicated by low numbers of
IgM- and IgG-memory B cells and increased numbers of CD21[low] B cells. Combined
homozygosity mapping and exome sequencing identified a biallelic splice-site mutation in
protein C kinase delta (*PRKCD*), causing absence of the corresponding protein product.
Consequently, phosphorylation of myristoylated alanine-rich C kinase substrate (MARCKS)
was decreased and mRNA levels of nuclear factor interleukin-6 (NF-IL6) and IL6 were
increased. Our study uncovers human PRKCD deficiency as a novel cause of common
variable immunodeficiency-like B cell deficiency with severe autoimmunity.

3.2.2 Introduction

Primary B cell immunodeficiencies (B-PID) constitute a heterogeneous group of immunodeficiencies characterized by defective production of antigen-specific antibodies and

predisposition to recurrent and severe infections (reviewed in[1]). A high proportion of patients display autoimmune features[2].

Fine-tuned B cell receptor (BCR) signaling is crucial for controlling immune homeostasis, as aberrant BCR signaling predisposes patients to autoimmunity (reviewed in[3]).

In the last decade, several Mendelian defects causing B-PID have been identified (reviewed in[3,4]). Nonetheless, the molecular etiology of these disorders remains elusive in the majority of patients. The advent of high-throughput genomic technologies will be instrumental in defining the spectrum of molecular aberrations underlying primary B cell deficiencies.

Here we investigated the molecular cause of a common variable immunodeficiency (CVID)-like B-PID with progressive B cell lymphopenia, immunoglobulin class switch defect, aberrant immunoglobulin levels and severe autoimmunity. Combined homozygosity mapping and exome sequencing identified a biallelic mutation in *PRKCD* encoding protein kinase C delta as the molecular cause of this novel PID.

3.2.3   Methods

A detailed description of all experimental methods can be found in the Supplement.

Subjects: This study has been approved by the ethics committee of the Medical University of Vienna, Austria. Biological material was obtained upon informed consent in accordance with the Declaration of Helsinki. The patient was followed up and treated at the Klinikum Wels-Griechirchen, St. Anna Kinderspital Vienna and the Department of Pediatrics and Adolescent Medicine of the Medical University of Vienna, Austria.

Flow cytometry-based immunophenotyping: Flow cytometry analysis of peripheral blood mononuclear cells was performed on a BD LSR Fortessa or BD FACS Calibur.

Genetic analysis: Sanger sequencing was performed according to standard methods; single nucleotide polymorphism (SNP)-based homozygosity mapping and exome sequencing were performed as described previously with minor modifications[5].

Immunoblot analysis: Immunoblot analyses were performed with the following antibodies: anti-human PRKCD (Cell Signaling, Germany), anti-phospho (clone D13E4) and total MARCKs (clone D88D11; both from Cell Signaling, Germany) and anti-GAPDH (clone 6C5; Santa Cruz Biotechnology, Germany).

Quantitative PCR (qPCR) analysis: mRNA levels of interleukin (*IL*)-*6* and nuclear factor (*NF*)-*IL6* in Epstein-Barr virus (EBV)-transformed B cells from the patient and his father upon stimulation with phorbol myristate acetate (PMA) were measured by qPCR analysis.

T *cell Vβ spectratyping*: TCR Vβ spectratyping was performed according to Pannetier *et al.*[6] with minor modifications.

3.2.4   Results and Discussion

Clinical and laboratory characterization

The index patient (now 12 years of age) was born to consanguineous parents (1st degree cousins) of Turkish origin (Supplementary Figure 1). His father was diagnosed with Behçet's disease and mild autoimmune thyreoiditis at 40 years of age. The mother is asymptomatic.

The patient's medical history is characterized by multifaceted manifestations of recurrent severe infections and autoimmunity as specified below.

Infections: From the first year of life onwards, the patient experienced repeated episodes of infections, including urinary tract infections, gastroenteritis, upper and lower respiratory tract infections as well as otitis media, prompting tonsillectomy and adenoidectomy within the first 4 years of life. Frequency and severity of infections normalized after commencement of immunoglobulin substitution at the age of 4 years.

Autoimmunity and immune dysregulation: The first manifestation of autoimmunity occurred at 15 months of age, when the patient presented with nephrotic syndrome. Renal biopsy revealed membranous glomerulonephritis (Figure 1A and Supplementary Figure 2). Partial remission was achieved upon steroid treatment with remaining mildly impaired renal function (low-grade proteinuria, hematuria; (Supplementary Table 1). By 3 years of age, hepatosplenomegaly (Supplementary Figure 3) and generalized lymphadenopathy became apparent, prompting in-depth diagnostic work-up, which revealed low-grade viremia of human herpes virus subtypes 6 and 7. Herpes viremia was transient while lymphadenopathy persisted. Several lymph node biopsies revealed nonspecific reactive follicular hyperplasia (Figure 1B). Bone marrow aspiration did not reveal any signs of malignancy (not shown). In the following years, additional manifestations of autoimmunity included relapsing polychondritis developed. Latent hypothyroidism was detected; organ-specific autoantibodies were absent. At the age of 8 years, aseptic endocarditis and pulmonary embolism were diagnosed and laboratory investigations suggested the diagnosis of anti-phospholipid syndrome (positivity of ANA, anti-dsDNA and anti-cardiolipin IgG antibodies; Supplementary Table 2), prompting anticoagulation therapy and low dose steroid-therapy.

Immunological work-up: Detailed laboratory evaluations were first performed after manifestation of glomerulonephritis at 15 months of age and revealed low IgG levels while levels of IgA and IgM were above normal range (Supplementary Figure 4). B cell studies showed reduction of CD19$^+$ B cells, decreased relative proportions of non class-switched (CD19$^+$CD27$^+$IgD$^+$) and class-switched (CD19$^+$CD27$^+$IgD$^-$) memory B cells as well as increased numbers of CD21^{low} B cells (Figure 1B-F and Supplementary Table 3). Longitudinal analyses showed progressive decline of total CD19$^+$ B cells (Figure 1D), increased relative proportion of CD21^{low} B cells (Figure 1E) and decreased frequencies of memory B cells (Figure 1F and G). T cell studies showed mildly decreased T cell proliferative responses (Supplementary Tables 2 and 3) without restriction of the TCR Vβ repertoire (Supplementary Figure 5). Impaired B cell function was suggested by absence of isohemagglutinins. Overall, findings were compatible with a CVID-like phenotype, though the formal criteria including decreased levels of at least two classes immunoglobulins[7] were not fulfilled.

Treatment: Due to recurrent respiratory tract infections including pneumonia, immunoglobulin G replacement was initiated at 4 years of age and led to decrease of infection frequency. At the age of 8 years, anti-CD20 therapy (two courses of 375mg/m^2 each) was performed to alleviate autoantibody production. Despite transient normalization of the previously increased IgM levels (Supplementary Figure 4), autoantibodies persisted. Since the age of 8 years, the patient has been under continuous treatment with mycophenolate-mofetil and low-dose steroids. Other treatment includes enalapril (angiotensin-converting enzyme inhibitor), anticoagulants, thyroid hormone replacement, and immunoglobulin replacement. With this treatment, the boy has a reasonably good quality of life, without need for hospitalization or intravenous antibiotics during the past three years.

Routine genetic investigation: Genetic work-up revealed no mutations in the *ICOS*, *BAFFR*, *TACI* and *FOXP3* genes, respectively. Surface expression of CD40/CD40ligand was normal. A heterozygous variant in *CTLA4* was discovered in both the index patient and his father (rs231775). Homozygosity for this variant has been associated with Graves's disease, rheumatoid arthritis and systemic lupus erythematous (SLE), while heterozygosity is associated with autoimmune thyreoiditis but not with SLE[8]. The clinical presentation of this patient with multiple features of immune dysregulation including glomerulonephritis, lymphadenopathy, relapsing polychondritis and antiphospholipid syndrome in the context of a CVID-like immune phenotype could not be reconciled with the heterozygous *CTLA4* variant alone. Thus, we initiated further genetic investigations to detect the molecular background of the patient's disease.

3.2.5   Mutation identification in the PRKCD gene

Given the consanguinity in the family, a monogenetic defect with autosomal recessive inheritance was assumed. To uncover the underlying genetic cause, we performed SNP array-based homozygosity mapping (Figure 2A and Supplementary Table 4) and exome sequencing (ES). Hits from ES were filtered for homozygous intervals present exclusively in the patient and validated by Sanger sequencing (Supplementary Figure 6, Supplementary Table 4). Only 2 of these hits showed perfect segregation with the disease: *UBXN1* (c. G686A, p. Thr229Met) and *PRKCD* (c.1352+1G>A), respectively (Figure 2B and Supplementary Figure 1).

While no obvious role for UBXN1 in the patient's disease pathogenesis could be recognized (see Supplement), PRKCD was considered a plausible candidate, since it has a well-established role in B cell signaling[9,10] and the corresponding *Prkcd-/-* knockout mouse exhibits various autoimmune manifestations together with generalized lymphadenopathy[11]. The murine model also shows splenic lymphocyte hyperproliferation[11], reminiscent of human autoimmune lymphoproliferative syndrome (ALPS)[12]. Western blot analysis revealed absence of PRKCD in the patient while expression was decreased in a heterozygous parent compared to a healthy control (Figure 2C). Lower expression in the heterozygous carrier does not seem to be sufficient to cause disease, as the parents do not present with the characteristic clinical features seen in the patient.

3.2.6   Functional consequences of PRKCD deficiency

PRKCD is a member of the protein kinase C (PKC) family critical for regulation of cell survival, proliferation and apoptosis (reviewed in[13]). In B lymphocytes, PRKCD is involved in BCR-mediated signaling downstream of BTK and PLCγ2 (reviewed in[9]). PRKCD is expected to have an essential function in B cell tolerance, as the corresponding knockout mouse shows immune-complex glomerulonephritis, splenomegaly and lymphadenopathy associated with B cell expansion and defective B cell tolerance to self-antigen[11]. Autoimmunity in *Prkcd-/-* mice has been linked to defective pro-apoptotic ERK signaling during B cell development[14]. Recently, *PLCγ2* mutations have been identified in CVID(-like) B cell deficiency with autoimmunity, highlighting the importance of this pathway for B cell homeostasis[15,16].

To assess functional consequences of PRKCD deficiency, expression of myristoylated alanine-rich C-kinase substrates (MARCKS), a major PKC target[17], was evaluated. Immunoblot analysis in EBV-immortalized patient B cell lines showed reduced total levels of

MARCKS despite contrary literature findings[18]. Importantly, MARCKS phosphorylation at Ser167/170, which is critical for translocation of MARCKS from the plasma membrane to the cytoplasm mediating reduction of cell proliferation[19], was abrogated in the patient (Figure 2D). Thus, deficiency of pMARCKS may be related to the lymphoproliferation in the patient[19].

Upon phosphorylation of NF-IL6 at Ser240 by PRKCD, DNA binding capability of NF-IL6 and consequently, IL6 production is markedly reduced[20]. Accordingly, we observed increased mRNA levels of *NF-IL6* and *IL6* in the PRKCD-deficient patient after PMA stimulation (Figure 2E), similar to hyperactive NF-IL6 signaling observed in *Prkcd -/-* mice[11].

In sum, we describe PRKCD deficiency as a novel primary, CVID-like B cell deficiency. The index patient of this study exhibited features of immune dysregulation including lympho-proliferation (splenomegaly, lymphadenopathy) and autoimmunity (glomerulonephritis, antiphospholipid syndrome, relapsing polychondritis) similar to the murine knockout model. However, neither peripheral B cell lymphopenia nor defective class switch observed in our patient were assessed in the mouse. It cannot be excluded that the known heterozygous variant in *CTLA4* in the patient may act as a disease-modifying factor. Future studies will need to comprehensively characterize the clinical and immunological phenotype in a cohort of PRKCD-deficient patients and further dissect the molecular pathophysiology of aberrant PRKCD-signaling in B cell homeostasis and autoimmunity.

3.2.7 Acknowledgments

We like to thank the family for their participation in this study and Georg Ebetsberger-Dachs, Ulrike Habeler and Christoph Male for clinical care and Karoly Lakatos for providing CT Scan pictures. We also thank Linda Stöger for help with qPCR analyses and Raphael Ott for technical assistance with library preparation for exome sequencing. We thank Ulrike Koermoeczi and Arno Rottal for expert technical assistance with flow cytometric analyses and Ciara Cleary for proofreading of the manuscript.

This work was supported by an intramural grant of CeMM Research Center for Molecular Medicine of the Austrian Academy of Sciences and the START Programme of the Austrian Science Fund (FWF): [Y595B13] (both to K.B.).

3.2.8 Author contributions

E.S., E.S.-V., S.K., S.B., N.K.P. and W.G. performed all experimental work except serial, routine immunological characterization performed by W.F.P.. W.E., H.B., A.H., F.E., M.G.S., K.A., W.H., A.P. and E.F.-W. provided clinical care and critically reviewed clinical and immunological patient data. L.M. and R.K. performed histopathological analyses. K.B. conceived this study with help from E.F.-W., planned, designed and interpreted experiments, provided laboratory resources, guided E.S., E.S.-V., S.K., S.B., N.K.P. and W.G., and wrote the initial draft of the manuscript with assistance from E.S., E.S-V., S.K., S.B., N.K.P. and E.F-W. All authors critically reviewed the manuscript and agreed to its publication. The authors declare that they have no relevant conflict of interest to disclose.

3.2.9   References

1.   Conley ME, Dobbs AK, Farmer DM, et al. Primary B cell immunodeficiencies: comparisons and contrasts. *Annual review of immunology.* 2009;27:199-227.

2.   Yong PF, Thaventhiran JE, Grimbacher B. "A rose is a rose is a rose," but CVID is Not CVID common variable immune deficiency (CVID), what do we know in 2011? *Adv Immunol.* 2011;111:47-107.

3.   van der Burg M, van Zelm MC, Driessen GJ, van Dongen JJ. New frontiers of primary antibody deficiencies. *Cell Mol Life Sci.* 2012;69(1):59-73.

4.   Al-Herz W, Bousfiha A, Casanova JL, et al. Primary immunodeficiency diseases: an update on the classification from the international union of immunological societies expert committee for primary immunodeficiency. *Front Immunol.* 2011;2:54.

5.   Salzer E, Daschkey S, Choo S, et al. Combined immunodeficiency with life-threatening EBV-associatedlymphoproliferative disorder in patients lacking functional CD27. *Haematologica.* 2012.

6.   Pannetier C, Even J, Kourilsky P. T-cell repertoire diversity and clonal expansions in normal and clinical samples. *Immunol Today.* 1995;16(4):176-181.

7.   Conley ME, Notarangelo LD, Etzioni A. Diagnostic criteria for primary immunodeficiencies. Representing PAGID (Pan-American Group for Immunodeficiency) and ESID (European Society for Immunodeficiencies). *Clinical immunology.* 1999;93(3):190-197.

8.   Gough SC, Walker LS, Sansom DM. CTLA4 gene polymorphism and autoimmunity. *Immunol Rev.* 2005;204:102-115.

9.   Guo B, Su TT, Rawlings DJ. Protein kinase C family functions in B-cell activation. *Curr Opin Immunol.* 2004;16(3):367-373.

10.   Zouali M, Sarmay G. B lymphocyte signaling pathways in systemic autoimmunity: implications for pathogenesis and treatment. *Arthritis Rheum.* 2004;50(9):2730-2741.

11.   Miyamoto A, Nakayama K, Imaki H, et al. Increased proliferation of B cells and auto-immunity in mice lacking protein kinase Cdelta. *Nature.* 2002;416(6883):865-869.

12.   Teachey DT. New advances in the diagnosis and treatment of autoimmune lymphoproliferative syndrome. *Curr Opin Pediatr.* 2012;24(1):1-8.

13.   Griner EM, Kazanietz MG. Protein kinase C and other diacylglycerol effectors in cancer. *Nature reviews Cancer.* 2007;7(4):281-294.

14.   Limnander A, Depeille P, Freedman TS, et al. STIM1, PKC-delta and RasGRP set a threshold for proapoptotic Erk signaling during B cell development. *Nature immunology.* 2011;12(5):425-433.

15.   Ombrello MJ, Remmers EF, Sun G, et al. Cold urticaria, immunodeficiency, and autoimmunity related to PLCG2 deletions. *The New England journal of medicine.* 2012;366(4):330-338.

16.   Zhou Q, Lee GS, Brady J, et al. A Hypermorphic Missense Mutation in PLCG2, Encoding Phospholipase Cgamma2, Causes a Dominantly Inherited Autoinflammatory Disease with Immunodeficiency. *American journal of human genetics.* 2012;91(4):713-720.

17.   Hartwig JH, Thelen M, Rosen A, Janmey PA, Nairn AC, Aderem A. MARCKS is an actin filament crosslinking protein regulated by protein kinase C and calcium-calmodulin. *Nature.* 1992;356(6370):618-622.

18.   Gallant C, You JY, Sasaki Y, Grabarek Z, Morgan KG. MARCKS is a major PKC-dependent regulator of calmodulin targeting in smooth muscle. *J Cell Sci.* 2005;118(Pt 16):3595-3605.

19.   Ramsden JJ. MARCKS: a case of molecular exaptation? *The international journal of biochemistry & cell biology.* 2000;32(5):475-479.

20. Trautwein C, van der Geer P, Karin M, Hunter T, Chojkier M. Protein kinase A and C site-specific phosphorylations of LAP (NF-IL6) modulate its binding affinity to DNA recognition elements. *The Journal of clinical investigation*. 1994;93(6):2554-2561.

21. Morbach H, Eichhorn EM, Liese JG, Girschick HJ. Reference values for B cell subpopulations from infancy to adulthood. *Clinical and experimental immunology*. 2010;162(2):271-279.

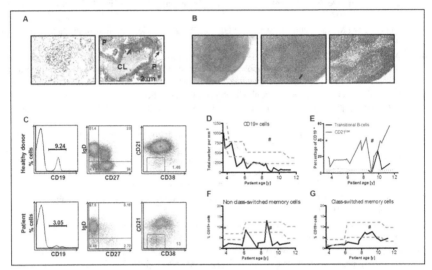

Figure 5: Clinical and immunological characterization of the index patient. First renal biopsy was performed at the age of 15 months. Granular deposition of IgG along the periphery of the capillary loops (upper panel) as seen in membranous nephropathy (MGN) was confirmed by transmission electron microscopy (TEM, lower panel) which showed electron dense deposits between basement membrane and podocytes (P) as well as deposits partially in resolution and incorporated by basement membrane material (arrows in lower panel) consistent with MGN stage I to III (CL; capillary loop) (A). Histopathological analysis of a lymph node biopsy revealed unspecific, reactive follicular hyperplasia (arrow) but not the characteristic lymph node changes of ALPS associated with *CD95/FAS* mutations (ALPS type 0/1a). The left and middle panel shows hematoxylin and eosin stains and the right panel shows anti-CD20 staining (B). Representative FACS plots illustrating the aberrant B cell phenotype including B cell lymphopenia, decreased IgM- and IgG memory B cells and increased numbers of CD21^{low} B cells are shown in (C). Longitudinal analysis illustrates progressive decrease of CD19+ B cells (D) and persistence of the aberrant distribution of B cell subsets (E-G). * marks the first episode of nephrotic syndrome, # indicates treatment with anti-CD20. The dotted lines indicate the age-related 25th and 75th percentile of the corresponding cells, respectively[22].

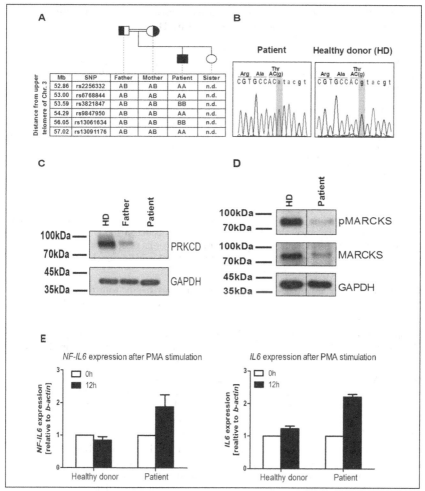

Figure 6: Identification of human PRKCD deficiency as a monogenetic B cell deficiency associated with autoimmunity. SNP-array based homozygosity mapping was performed and revealed several homozygous candidate intervals, including an interval on Chromosome 3p21.31 (A). Sanger sequencing validated a splice site mutation in *PRKCD*, encoding for protein kinase C delta, which was homozygous in the patient (B). Western blot analysis showed absent expression of the corresponding protein product in the patient, compared with decreased expression in the heterozygous father and normal expression in a healthy control (C). Western blot analysis showed defective phosphorylation of myristoylated alanine-rich C kinase substrate (MARCKS), a downstream target of PRKCD (D). Quantitative PCR analysis (qPCR) showed hyperactive NF-IL6 signaling upon stimulation using PMA, as indicated by increased mRNA levels of *NF-IL6* and *IL6*, respectively (E).

3.3 Early-onset inflammatory bowel disease and common variable ...
immunodeficiency–like disease caused by IL-21 deficiency

Elisabeth Salzer,[1] Aydan Kansu,[2] Heiko Sic,[3] Peter Majek,[1] Aydan Ikinciogullari,[4][SEP]Figen E. Dogu,[4] Nina Kathrin Prengemann,[1] Elisangela Santos-Valente,[1] Winfried F. Pickl,[5] Ivan Bilic,[1] Sol A Ban,[1] Zarife Kuloglu,[2] Arzu Meltem Demir,[2] Arzu Ensari,[6] Jacques Colinge,[1] Marta Rizzi,[3] Hermann Eibel,[3] and Kaan Boztug[1,7]

[1]CeMM Research Center for Molecular Medicine of the Austrian Academy of Sciences, Vienna; the Departments of [2]Pediatric Gastroenterology, [4]Pediatric Immunology, and [6]Pathology, Ankara University; [3]the Center for Chronic Immuno- deficiency, University Medical Center, Freiburg; [5]the Christian Doppler Laboratory for Immunomodulation and Institute of Immunology, Center for Pathophysiology, Infectiology and Immunology, and [7]the Department of Pediatrics and Adolescent Medicine, Medical University of Vienna.

3.3.1 Abstract

Background: Alterations of the immune homeostasis in the gut may result in the development of inflammatory bowel disease (IBD). Recently, Mendelian forms of IBD have been discovered as exemplified by deficiency of interleukin 10 or its receptor subunits. In addition, other types of primary immunodeficiency disorders (PIDs) may be associated with intestinal inflammation as one of their leading clinical presentations.

Objective: We here investigated a large consanguineous family with three children who presented with early-onset inflammatory bowel disease within the first year of life, leading to death in infancy in two of them.

Methods: Homozyosity mapping combined with exome sequencing was performed to identify the molecular cause of the disorder. Functional experiments were performed to assess the impact of the identified variant in *IL21* on the immune system.

Results: A homozygous mutation in *IL21* was discovered which showed perfect segregation with the disease. Deficiency of IL21 resulted in reduced numbers of circulating CD19[+] B cells including IgM[+] naïve and class-switched IgG memory B cells with a concomitant increase in transitional B cells. *In vitro* assays demonstrated that mutant IL21[Leu49Pro] failed to induce STAT3 phosphorylation and immunoglobulin class switch recombination.

Conclusion: Our study uncovers IL21 deficiency as a novel cause of early-onset inflammatory bowel disease in humans, accompanied by defects in B cell development similar to those found in common variable immunodeficiency. Inflammatory bowel disease may mask an underlying primary immunodeficiency as illustrated here with IL21 deficiency.

3.3.2 Introduction

A tightly regulated balance of the immune system is critical for immune homeostasis and, if altered, may be responsible for the development of inflammatory bowel disease (IBD)[1]. Genome-wide association studies to identify genetic factors of complex IBD traits have suggested that both genetic and environmental factors contribute to the disease[2-4]. The majority of susceptibility loci identified have revealed genes important in immunological processes[5]. More recently, early-onset Mendelian forms of IBD have been recognized, as illustrated by the discovery of Interleukin-10 (-receptor) deficiency[6].

Intriguingly, patients suffering from various primary immunodeficiency disorders (PIDs) can also exhibit intestinal inflammation as one of their leading symptoms[7]. For instance, qualitative or quantitative neutrophil defects, such as chronic granulomatous disease (CGD)[8] or G6PC3 deficiency[9], have been associated with chronic intestinal inflammation. In addition, patients with partial T cell deficiency, Wiscott-Aldrich syndrome[10, 11], LRBA deficiency[12] or defects in the development of regulatory T cells[13] may present with colitis. Similarly, primary B cell deficiencies including the subgroup of common variable immunodeficiencies (CVIDs) frequently display an IBD-like phenotype[14, 15]. These observations indicate that multiple immunopathological processes can result in IBD and point to the gastrointestinal tract as a particularly vulnerable site for aberrations of immune homeostasis. We here describe IL21 deficiency as a novel primary immunodeficiency which may associate a common variable immunodeficiency (CVID)-like B cell deficiency with early-onset IBD.

3.3.3 Methods

Patient and Ethics: This study has been approved by the responsible local ethics committee. Biological material was obtained upon informed consent in accordance with the Declaration of Helsinki. The patient was followed up and treated at the Departments of Immunology and Gastroenterology, respectively, at Ankara University in Turkey.

Flow cytometry-based immunophenotyping: Flow cytometric analyses were performed on a BD LSR Fortessa, BD FACS Canto or BD FACS Calibur. In brief, peripheral blood mono-nuclear cells (PBMCs) from the patient and a healthy control were isolated using Ficoll density gradient centrifugation and stained for 20 minutes at 4°C with mouse anti-human antibodies: CD3-APC-H7 (clone SK7, BD-Biosciences, Vienna, Austria), CD4-APC (clone RPA-T4, BD-Biosciences), CD8-V500 (clone RPA-T8, BD-Biosciences), CD19-PerCPCy5.5 (clone HIB19, eBioscience, Vienna, Austria), CD21-PE (clone B-ly4, BD-Biosciences), CD27-Brilliant violet (clone M-T271, BD-Biosciences), CD38-PECy7 (clone HIT2, BD-Biosciences), IgD-FITC (clone IA6-2, BD-Biosciences) and IgM-APC (clone G20-127, BD-Biosciences), TCRab (FITC clone WT31, BD-Biosciences), TCRgd (PE, clone 11F2, BD-Biosciences). Activation of B cells, in-depth B cell phenotyping and stimulation were carried out as published previously[16-18].

Genetic analyses: Genomic DNA sequencing of *IL10*, *IL10RA* and *IL10RB* was performed according to standard methods (see Supplementary Methods for details). Single nucleotide polymorphism (SNP)-based homozygosity mapping and exome sequencing were performed as described previously[19] with minor modifications (Supplementary Methods).

Recombinant protein production: Recombinant protein production using the HEK-EBNA system was carried out as described previously[20, 21]. In brief, HEK-EBNA cells were seeded in a 10 cm dish in complete DMEM (PAA, Invitrogen, Vienna Austria) and transfected with 5 µg of vectors encoding N-terminally His-tagged IL21[wildtype] and IL21[Leu49Pro]. Transfected cells were selected with complete DMEM containing 1 µg/ml puromycine (Sigma Aldrich, Vienna, Austria). Once confluence was reached, cells were set on serum-free DMEM to initiate IL21 production. Supernatants were collected after 1 week, filter sterilized and frozen at -80°C. To test successful IL21 production, trichloroacetic acid precipitation was performed at -20°C over night. Subsequently, proteins were washed with 80% aceton and 100% acetone once each, air-dried and resuspended in Lämmli-buffer. Equal volumes of sterile-filtered super-natants were loaded on a 12% acrylamide gel and the membrane was probed against the His-tag of the produced proteins to assess equal production and stability of wildtype and mutant

IL21 protein, respectively (Supplementary Figure 4B). Subsequently, stimulation experiments were carried out using equal volumes of supernatants and thus equal amounts of mutant and wiltype IL21, respectively.

*Stimulation of Jurkat cells:*_5x10^6 Jurkat cells per condition were serum starved to reduce global phosphorylation levels and stimulated with equal volumes of IL21^{wildtype}, IL21^{Leu49Pro} or 10 ng/ml commercially available recombinant IL21 (eBiosciences, Vienna, Austria), respectively, for 30 minutes. Cells were washed once with cold phosphate buffered saline, spun down and the pellet was snap frozen in liquid nitrogen. Protein was isolated using cell lysis buffer containing 20 mM Tris (pH7.5), 150 mM NaCl, 2 mM EDTA, 1% TritonX-100 (pH7.1) and complete protease inhibitor cocktail (Sigma Aldrich). Samples were run on an 8% acrylamide gel at constant voltage of 110V for two hours and blotted at 350 mA for 1.5 h. Membranes were blocked using 5% BSA-tris buffered saline-containing 0.05% Tween (Sigma Aldrich) and incubated with the respective antibodies over night at 4°C.

*Immunoblot analysis:*_The primary antibodies used for western blot analysis were rabbit anti-human STAT3, pSTAT3 (Tyr701, 58D6; both from Cell Signaling, Frankfurt am Main, Germany). Primary antibodies directed against His (AD1.1.10) and a mouse anti-human GAPDH antibody (clone 6C5; both from Santa Cruz Biotechnology, Heidelberg, Germany) were used. Horseradish peroxidase (HRP)-conjugated goat anti-rabbit (Bio-rad, Vienna, Austria) and goat anti-mouse (BD-Biosciences) secondary antibodies were detected using a chemiluminescent substrate (Amersham ECL Prime Western Blotting Detection Reagent, GE Life Sciences, Vienna, Austria). Detection was performed by autoradiography using :

*T cell Proliferation Analysis:*_T cell proliferation assays were carried out as described previously[19].

*T cell Vb spectratyping:*_TCR Vb spectratyping was performed according to Pannetier *et al.*[22] with minor modifications as described previously[19] (see supplementary information).

*In silico analyses of IL21:*_In brief, molecular dynamics simulations of wildtype and mutant IL-21 were performed using the coarse-gained model FREADDY[23] implemented in MOIL[23, 24] molecular modeling package with different degrees of flexibility. All simulations predicted the same qualitative behaviour. For details please see supplementary information.

3.3.4   Results

Clinical characterization of the patient

The index patient (currently 11 years of age) was born to healthy Turkish consanguineous parents (1st degree cousins). Two out of eight of the patient's siblings died of severe diarrhea before 1 year of age (2 months and 8 months of age, respectively). The index patient's disease is characterized by both early-onset inflammatory bowel disease and a CVID-like immunodeficiency as specified below.

Inflammatory bowel disease: The patient initially presented to the hospital at 2 months of age with persistent, mucoid, non-bloody diarrhea and recurrent oral aphtous ulcers. Additionally, he exhibited signs of chronic disease such as fatigue and failure to thrive with body weight being constantly below the third percentile (not shown). He did not show any general skin lesions, perianal lesions, fistulas, uveitis or signs of arthritis, respectively. During the following years, diarrhea persisted and malnutrition as well as finger clubbing became apparent. Microbiology analyses feces for *Cryptosporidium, Giardia lamblia*, rotavirus and adenovirus returned negative. Colonoscopy revealed macroscopically a loss of vascular pattern, mucosal erythema as well as edema and aphtous ulcers (Figure 1A). Biopsies showed eosinophil and neutrophil infiltration, focal cryptitis, focal active colitis as well as non-caseating granuloma, as seen in typical Crohn's disease (Figure 1B). As a part of a local study protocol for early-onset IBD patients, magnetic resonance cholangiopancreaticography (MRCP) was performed which did not reveal any abnormalities. The patient was evaluated for familial mediterranean fever, therefore exons 2 and 10 of *MEVF* were sequenced and a heterozygous carrier status of a common mutation (p. Met694Val) was detected. Based on colonoscopic and histologic findings, the patient was diagnosed with Crohn's disease. Treatment with mesalazine, omega-3 fatty acids and supplementary enteral feeding was initiated but chronic diarrhea persisted. The patient, now 11 years of age, is still malnourished with body weight persistently below the 3rd percentile (not shown).

Immunodeficiency: At the age of four, the patient was referred for assessment of a potential underlying immunodeficiency. Laboratory examinations revealed increased IgE levels (119 kU/ml) while immunoglobulin G (IgG) levels (338 mg/dl) and isohemagglutins were reduced (titer 1:2) (Table 1). In retrospect, the patient experienced recurrent and severe upper and lower respiratory tract infections at an unusually high frequency from the age of one year onwards. Since not all criteria for CVID diagnosis were met as IgG was the sole type of immunoglobulin which was reduced (Table1), the patient was diagnosed with a CVID-like immunodeficiency[28, 29]. Intravenous immunoglobulin replacement together with prophylactic trimetoprim-sulfamethoxazole therapy was started. At present, the patient exhibits signs of severe chronic pulmonary infections such as finger clubbing.

Detailed immunological work up: The patient was vaccinated according to general recommendations, receiving vaccinations against Bacillus Calmette-Guérin (BCG), Hepatitis-B Virus (HBV), Diptheria-Pertussis-Tetantus-Polio as well as measles. Anti-HBV surface antigen (HBs) titers were found borderline low and antibody titers against BCG were negative. He was also evaluated for auto-antibodies such as anti-neutrophil antibodies, anti-neutrophil cytoplasmic antibodoes, thyreoglobulin antibodies, anti-gliadin IgA and IgG which were negative at 9 years of life. PCR-based evaluation for cytomegalovirus and human immunodeficiency virus was negative. In order to exclude known hereditary immuno-deficiency syndromes, CD40, CD40L and FOXP3 expression was evaluated using flow cytometry and found to be normal (data not shown). *Cryptosporidium* in feces was tested negative at the age of 6 years and 9 years, respectively. To assess potential chronic granulomatous disease, neutrophil oxidative burst assays were performed at the age of 5 years but did not show any abnormalities (data not shown). Due to the severity and early onset of inflammatory bowel disease in this patient *IL10*, *IL10RA* and *IL10RB* genes were sequenced but no mutation could be detected (data not shown).

Mutation identification in the *IL21* gene

Given the consanguinity in the family and the occurrence of early-onset IBD in 3 out of 8 siblings, a monogenetic defect with autosomal recessive inheritance was suspected (Figure 1C). Single nucleotide polymorphism (SNP) array-based homozygosity mapping (Supple-mentary Table 1 and 2) and exome sequencing (ES) were then performed to identify the underlying genetic defect. Hits from ES were filtered for homozygous intervals present in the patient and validated by capillary sequencing (Supplementary methods and results). A total of 2 hits were validated which showed perfect segregation among the core family members. No obvious role for the variant in *ENPEP* in the disease of the patient could be detected (see supplementary information). The second hit, a homozygous mutation in *IL21* (c.T147C, p.Leu49Pro), showed perfect segregation under the assumption of autosomal recessive inheritance with full penetrance and could not be detected in existing single nucleotide polymorphism databases such as ENSEMBL, dbSNP and UCSC (date of accession: December, 30th, 2013) (Figures 1C and 1D). In light of the marked IBD phenotype in all 3 affected individuals in this family, we intersected exome data from the patient with known SNPs predisposing for inflammatory bowel disease (taken from http://www.genome.gov/page.cfm?pageid=26525384#searchForm). However, no known SNPs in *IL23R* or *NOD2*, associated with inflammatory bowel disease could be detected in the patient (data not shown).

The mutated residue IL21^{Leu49} is highly conserved throughout evolution (Figure 1E). Prediction of the protein folding stability of the IL21^{Leu49Pro} variant using the CUPSAT protein stability analysis tool[24] suggested that any change of IL21^{Leu49} would reduce the stability of the native state. Notably, the strongest destabilization of the native state of the protein folding was predicted by changing IL21^{Leu49} to proline (Supplementary Table 3). CUPSAT predictions were supported by coarse-grained molecular dynamics simulations of IL21^{wildtype} and IL21^{Leu49Pro}. In the simulation of IL21^{wildtype}, IL21^{Leu49} remains fully buried within the protein core, whereas the protein core of the IL21^{Leu49Pro} mutant is predicted to be unstable in the original orientation, undergoing a transition to the outer side of the helix A into the gap between helices A and C (Figure 1F) within 10 ns (Figure 1G). This transition is accompanied by an extension of the alpha helical part of the helix A (the C-terminal end of the A is a 3_{10} helix in the wildtype fold) and slight modification of the relative position of the helices A and C (Figure 1F). As the crystal structure of IL21 bound to the IL21R (PDB id 3TGX) demonstrates that helices A and C of IL21 are critical for receptor binding and initiation of signaling of the JAK-Stat signaling cascade[30], the predicted conformational change caused by the *IL21*^{Leu49Pro} mutation most likely lowers the affinity of IL21 binding to IL21R.

Functional consequences of IL21 deficiency

Based on the hypothesis that the patient's disease is most likely caused by defective IL21 function that impairs adaptive immunity[31,32] a more detailed analysis of the patient's immunological phenotype was performed. Compared to healthy controls, the patient had fewer circulating CD19$^+$ B cells, almost no CD19$^+$CD27$^+$IgD$^+$ marginal zone-like and CD19$^+$CD27$^+$IgD$^-$ class-switched memory B cells (Figure 2A, Supplementary Figure 1), resulting in a relative increase in CD19$^+$CD38^{hi}CD23$^-$ transitional B cells (Figure 2B). Accordingly, very few IgG$^+$ or IgA$^+$ cells were detected in peripheral blood of the patient compared to control (Figure 2C). Analysis of T cell subsets revealed normal relative proportions of CD3$^+$CD4$^+$ T-helper cell and CD3$^+$CD8$^+$ cytotoxic T cell subsets (not shown), but an increase in CD3$^+$ TCRgd cells (Supplementary Figure 2). The cell receptor Vb repertoire was found to be polyclonal (Supplementary Figure 3) and cell proliferation induced by various stimuli was found to be normal (Figure 2D, left panel) except for tetanus toxoid stimulation despite the fact that the patient has a history of tetanus toxoid vaccinations (Figure 2D, right panel).

IL21^{Leu49Pro} fails to induce IL21R signaling, proliferation and activation of B cells

The effects of Leu49Pro on the activity of the cytokine were analyzed by comparing *in vitro* B and T cell responses induced by equal amounts of recombinant mutant (IL21^{Leu49Pro}) or wildtype protein (IL21^{wildtype}) produced in HEK-EBNA cells (Supplementary Figure 4). To exclude donor-dependent differences in T cell responses, a Jurkat T cell line was used to test STAT3 phosphorylation. Stimulation with either commercially available recombinant IL21 (IL21^{rec}) or IL21^{wildtype} phosphorylated the STAT3 tyrosine residue 705, whereas IL21^{Leu49Pro}

failed to induce STAT3 phosphorylation at this position (Figure 3A). Differences between IL21^{wildtype} and IL21^{Leu49Pro} in activating B cells were tested on normal donor cord blood-derived B cells. Proliferation of total CD19$^+$ (Figure 3B) and of transitional cord blood-derived CD19$^+$ B cells (Figure 3C), as well as proliferation of memory and plasmablast subsets (Supplementary Figure 5), were strongly decreased upon activation with mutant IL21^{Leu49Pro}.

IL21-deficient B cells can be activated and undergo class-switch recombination

To exclude intrinsic defects affecting the patient's B cells, PBMCs were stimulated for three days with CD40L and IL21, or alternatively with CD40L and IL4, and tested for the expression of activation markers CD69, CD86 and CD95 and class-switch recombination indicated by surface expression of IgG and IgA, respectively.

As expected, the expression pattern of the activation markers was normal in the B cells of the patient (Figure 4A). Similar to control B cells, they proliferated and differentiated into IgG$^+$/IgA$^+$ cells in response to IL21, strongly suggesting that the B cells of the patient have an intact capacity to develop into plasma cells and memory B cells in response to IL21R signaling (Figure 4B).

3.3.5   Discussion

Combining homozygosity mapping with exome sequencing, we uncovered IL21 deficiency as novel monogenetic cause of severe, early-onset inflammatory bowel disease associated with a CVID-like primary immunodeficiency. IL21 belongs to type I cytokine family and acts on many cells of the hematopoietic system[33]. IL21 is predominantly produced by antigen-activated CD4$^+$ T cells and activated B-helper neutrophils[34]. B-helper neutrophils secrete IL21 to promote T cell-independent B cell responses against microbes[34]. Therefore, our finding that IL21 deficiency causes early-onset IBD suggests that IL21 plays a critical role in the cooperation between the innate and adaptive immunity in the gut.

IL21R is expressed by T, B and NK cells, subsets of myeloid cells as well as keratinocytes[35-38]. IL21 binding to IL21R induces primarily STAT1 and STAT3 phosphorylation[32]. It therefore differs from other type I cytokines such as IL2, IL7, IL9 and IL15, since these cytokines induce STAT3 and STAT5 activation, whereas IL4 activates STAT6[39, 40]. IL21 does not seem to influence T$_H$1 or T$_H$2 polarization in CD4$^+$ T cells[41, 42], but it seems to be critical for proliferation and activation of both naïve and memory CD8$^+$ T cells[42]. In NK cells, IL21 contributes to the phenotypic and functional maturation by inducing the expression of killer-immunoglobulin-like receptors, perforin expression and interferon gamma secretion[43, 44]. In CD40L-activated B cells, IL21 strongly promotes proliferation, immunoglobulin class switch recombination and Ig secretion[41, 45], while inhibiting the IL4-driven induction of germ-line transcripts from the IgE constant region[46, 47]. Accordingly, *Il21r-/-* knockout mice show dysgammaglobulinemia characterized by low IgG$_1$ levels but higher IgE levels[41]. In humans, IL21R deficiency has recently been reported to result in primary immunodeficiency characterized by defective B cell class switch, aberrant T cell cytokine production and NK cell cytotoxicity[48].

Surprisingly, in contrast to the patients reported with IL21R deficiency, the IL21-deficient patient presented here developed early-onset inflammatory bowel disease, which masked primary immunodeficiency found at a later age. In addition, two of the patient's siblings died of IBD within the first year of life, underlining the consistency of early-onset IBD presentation in this pedigree. Furthermore, the patient has to date not shown any signs of cholangitis and was negative for *Cryptosporidium* infection, one of the most striking observations in 3 out of 4 of the described IL21R-deficient patients[48]. However, two out of the four patients with IL21R deficiency also presented with diarrhea, which was possibly attributed to *Cryptosporidium* infection and therefore not thought to be a primary cause of defective IL21R-dependent signaling. *Cryptospridium* infections are common in patients with combined immunodeficiencies[49] and may have altered the clinical features of the immunodeficiency in the reported IL21R-deficient patients. In addition, we cannot exclude underlying differences in the gut microbiota, which are essential non genetic-players in the development of inflammatory bowel disease[50, 51]. Future studies will need to address the complex interplay of the microbiome on disease course of monogenetically determined immunodeficiency disorders.

The primary immunodeficiency caused by mutation in the *IL21* gene was characterized by reduced relative numbers of B cells and dramatically reduced class-switched memory B cell populations, increased IgE levels and hypogammaglobulinemia in peripheral blood. These findings are in line with the observations from murine models[52] and human IL21R deficiency[48]. Although proliferation of IL21$^{\text{Leu49Pro}}$-expressing T cells appeared normal upon stimulation with several common stimuli, stimulation with specific agents such as tetanus toxoid illustrated specific defects in T cell proliferation, thus recapitulating the findings described for IL21R deficiency[48].

Interestingly, approximately 20% of CVID patients develop autoimmunity which often results in colitis and is associated with severely increased morbidity[14]. It has been hypothesized that IL21 has immunosuppressive activities by inducing IL10 secretion[53]. Similar to IL10 or IL10R deficiency, IBD in the IL21-deficient patient manifested in the first year of life and was characterized by a severe phenotype[6, 11, 54, 55]. It has been shown previously that synergistic stimulation of bone marrow- or spleen-derived NK cells with IL21 and IL2 or IL15 leads to increased IL10 secretion, suggesting that the IBD might be due to decreased IL10 secretion caused by IL21 deficiency[39]. Nevertheless, the molecular mechanisms how IL21 deficiency leads to gut inflammation remain elusive.

IL21 has emerged as a critical cytokine regulating multiple arms of the immune system (reviewed in [32]). More recently, interfering with IL21 signaling has been proposed as a treatment option for various autoimmune diseases including systemic lupus erythematosus[56] and rheumatoid diseases[57, 58]. However, our observation that lack of functional IL21 is associated with an immunodeficiency with considerable morbidity raises an important concern for such therapeutic strategies.

In principle, IL21 deficiency may be amenable to allogeneic hematopoietic stem cell transplantation (aHSCT) to correct for the disease[6, 54], however, given the currently stable clinical condition, this has not been performed in the patient to date but remains an option for the future. In contrast to IL21R deficiency, treatment with recombinant IL21 may represent an alternative, experimental strategy for treatment of IL21 deficiency in a similar manner as has been proposed for metastatic cancer including metastatic melanoma[59] and renal cell carcinoma[60,61, 62]. This may be particularly attractive for scenarios when the patient's clinical status is incompatible with aHSCT.

In conclusion, here we identify deficiency of IL21 as a novel cause of primary immunodeficiency and early-onset inflammatory bowel disease, thereby further underlining the critical importance of tight control of immune homeostasis for inflammatory processes in the gut. Future studies will show whether targeting the affected pathways is a therapeutic option for IL21 deficiency and related disorders.

3.3.6 Acknowledgments

We would like to thank the family for their participation in this study and all clinicians who helped to manage the patient through the course of the disease. We also thank Linda Stöger for exclusion of coding mutations in *IL10, IL10RA and IL10RB* as well as Raphael Ott for assistance with library preparation for exome sequencing and Cecilia Domínguez Conde for critical proofreading of the manuscript. In addition we would like to thank Frank Zaucke and his team for providing the HEK-EBNA system for recombinant protein production. This study has been supported by funding from the Austrian Science Fund (FWF) grant number P24999 to K.B. and the German ministry for Research and Technology, the German Cancer Research fund (grant 1098935, both to H.E.) as well as German Federal Ministry of Education and Research (BMBF 01 EO 0803) to M.R.

3.3.7 Author Contributions

E.S. performed all experimental work except for B cell class switch and activation assays which were performed by H.S., H.E. and M.R. as well as T cell proliferation assays which were performed by W.F.P., A.K., A.I., F.E.D., Z.K., A.M.D. and A.E. provided clinical care of the patient performed routine clinical interventions. P.M. performed computational modeling and *in silico* prediction algorithms. S.A.B. performed TCR Vβ spectratyping of the patient and N.K.P. and E.S.-V. assisted in experimental procedures and performed SNP chip based homozygosity mapping. K.B. conceived this study, provided laboratory resources and together with E.S. planned, designed and interpreted experiments. E.S. and K.B. wrote the first draft and the revised version of the manuscript with input from K.B., A.K., A.I., F.D. and H.E. All authors critically reviewed the manuscript and agreed to its publication.

The authors declare that they have no relevant conflict of interest to disclose.

3.3.8 References

1. Qin J, Li R, Raes J, Arumugam M, Burgdorf KS, Manichanh C, et al. A human gut microbial gene catalogue established by metagenomic sequencing. Nature 2010; 464:59-65.

2. Brant SR. Update on the heritability of inflammatory bowel disease: the importance of twin studies. Inflamm Bowel Dis 2011; 17:1-5.

3. Cho JH. The genetics and immunopathogenesis of inflammatory bowel disease. Nat Rev Immunol 2008; 8:458-66.

4. Xavier RJ, Podolsky DK. Unravelling the pathogenesis of inflammatory bowel disease. Nature 2007; 448:427-34.

5. Khor B, Gardet A, Xavier RJ. Genetics and pathogenesis of inflammatory bowel disease. Nature 2011; 474:307-17.

6. Glocker EO, Kotlarz D, Boztug K, Gertz EM, Schaffer AA, Noyan F, et al. Inflammatory bowel disease and mutations affecting the interleukin-10 receptor. N Engl J Med 2009; 361:2033-45.

7. Arkwright PD, Abinun M, Cant AJ. Autoimmunity in human primary immunodeficiency diseases. Blood 2002; 99:2694-702.

8.   Marks DJ, Miyagi K, Rahman FZ, Novelli M, Bloom SL, Segal AW. Inflammatory bowel disease in CGD reproduces the clinicopathological features of Crohn's disease. Am J Gastroenterol 2009; 104:117-24.

9.   Begin P, Patey N, Mueller P, Rasquin A, Sirard A, Klein C, et al. Inflammatory Bowel Disease and T cell Lymphopenia in G6PC3 Deficiency. Journal of clinical immunology 2012.

10.   Dupuis-Girod S, Medioni J, Haddad E, Quartier P, Cavazzana-Calvo M, Le Deist F, et al. Autoimmunity in Wiskott-Aldrich syndrome: risk factors, clinical features, and outcome in a single-center cohort of 55 patients. Pediatrics 2003; 111:e622-7.

11.   Glocker E, Grimbacher B. Inflammatory bowel disease: is it a primary immunodeficiency? Cell Mol Life Sci 2012; 69:41-8.

12.   Alangari A, Alsultan A, Adly N, Massaad MJ, Kiani IS, Aljebreen A, et al. LPS-responsive beige-like anchor (LRBA) gene mutation in a family with inflammatory bowel disease and combined immunodeficiency. J Allergy Clin Immunol 2012; 130:481-8 e2.

13.   Barzaghi F, Passerini L, Bacchetta R. Immune dysregulation, polyendocrinopathy, enteropathy, x-linked syndrome: a paradigm of immunodeficiency with autoimmunity. Front Immunol 2012; 3:211.

14.   Bussone G, Mouthon L. Autoimmune manifestations in primary immune deficiencies. Autoimmun Rev 2009; 8:332-6.

15.   Agarwal S, Smereka P, Harpaz N, Cunningham-Rundles C, Mayer L. Characterization of immunologic defects in patients with common variable immunodeficiency (CVID) with intestinal disease. Inflamm Bowel Dis 2011; 17:251-9.

16.   Warnatz K, Schlesier M. Flowcytometric phenotyping of common variable immunodeficiency. Cytometry B Clin Cytom 2008; 74:261-71.

17.   Warnatz K, Salzer U, Rizzi M, Fischer B, Gutenberger S, Bohm J, et al. B-cell activating factor receptor deficiency is associated with an adult-onset antibody deficiency syndrome in humans. Proc Natl Acad Sci U S A 2009; 106:13945-50.

18.   Kienzler AK, Rizzi M, Reith M, Nutt SL, Eibel H. Inhibition of human B-cell development into plasmablasts by histone deacetylase inhibitor valproic acid. J Allergy Clin Immunol 2013; 131:1695-9.

19.   Salzer E, Daschkey S, Choo S, Gombert M, Santos-Valente E, Ginzel S, et al. Combined immunodeficiency with life-threatening EBV-associated lymphoproliferative disorder in patients lacking functional CD27. Haematologica 2013; 98:473-8.

20.   Agarwal P, Zwolanek D, Keene DR, Schulz JN, Blumbach K, Heinegard D, et al. Collagen XII and XIV, new partners of cartilage oligomeric matrix protein in the skin extracellular matrix suprastructure. J Biol Chem 2012; 287:22549-59.

21.   Bechtel M, Keller MV, Bloch W, Sasaki T, Boukamp P, Zaucke F, et al. Different domains in nidogen-1 and nidogen-2 drive basement membrane formation in skin organotypic cocultures. FASEB J 2012; 26:3637-48.

22.   Pannetier C, Even J, Kourilsky P. T-cell repertoire diversity and clonal expansions in normal and clinical samples. Immunol Today 1995; 16:176-81.

23.   ELBER R. MOIL: A Program for simulations of macromolecules. 1995; Computer Physics Communications:159-89.

24.   Parthiban V, Gromiha MM, Schomburg D. CUPSAT: prediction of protein stability upon point mutations. Nucleic Acids Res 2006; 34:W239-42.

25.   Bondensgaard K, Breinholt J, Madsen D, Omkvist DH, Kang L, Worsaae A, et al. The existence of multiple conformers of interleukin-21 directs engineering of a superpotent analogue. J Biol Chem 2007; 282:23326-36.

26.   Zhang Y, Skolnick J. Scoring function for automated assessment of protein structure template quality. Proteins 2004; 57:702-10.

27. Pettersen EF, Goddard TD, Huang CC, Couch GS, Greenblatt DM, Meng EC, et al. UCSF Chimera--a visualization system for exploratory research and analysis. J Comput Chem 2004; 25:1605-12.

28. Conley ME, Dobbs AK, Farmer DM, Kilic S, Paris K, Grigoriadou S, et al. Primary B cell immunodeficiencies: comparisons and contrasts. Annu Rev Immunol 2009; 27:199-227.

29. Yong PF, Thaventhiran JE, Grimbacher B. "A rose is a rose is a rose," but CVID is Not CVID common variable immune deficiency (CVID), what do we know in 2011? Adv Immunol 2011; 111:47-107.

30. Hamming OJ, Kang L, Svensson A, Karlsen JL, Rahbek-Nielsen H, Paludan SR, et al. Crystal structure of interleukin-21 receptor (IL-21R) bound to IL-21 reveals that sugar chain interacting with WSXWS motif is integral part of IL-21R. J Biol Chem 2012; 287:9454-60.

31. Skak K, Kragh M, Hausman D, Smyth MJ, Sivakumar PV. Interleukin 21: combination strategies for cancer therapy. Nat Rev Drug Discov 2008; 7:231-40.

32. Leonard WJ, Spolski R. Interleukin-21: a modulator of lymphoid proliferation, apoptosis and differentiation. Nat Rev Immunol 2005; 5:688-98.

33. Lichtmann AHAAK. Cellular and Molecular Immunology (5th Edition). Philadelphia: Saunders; 2003.

34. Puga I, Cols M, Barra CM, He B, Cassis L, Gentile M, et al. B cell-helper neutrophils stimulate the diversification and production of immunoglobulin in the marginal zone of the spleen. Nat Immunol 2012; 13:170-80.

35. Parrish-Novak J, Dillon SR, Nelson A, Hammond A, Sprecher C, Gross JA, et al. Interleukin 21 and its receptor are involved in NK cell expansion and regulation of lymphocyte function. Nature 2000; 408:57-63.

36. Brandt K, Bulfone-Paus S, Foster DC, Ruckert R. Interleukin-21 inhibits dendritic cell activation and maturation. Blood 2003; 102:4090-8.

37. Brandt K, Bulfone-Paus S, Jenckel A, Foster DC, Paus R, Ruckert R. Interleukin-21 inhibits dendritic cell-mediated T cell activation and induction of contact hypersensitivity in vivo. J Invest Dermatol 2003; 121:1379-82.

38. Distler JH, Jungel A, Kowal-Bielecka O, Michel BA, Gay RE, Sprott H, et al. Expression of interleukin-21 receptor in epidermis from patients with systemic sclerosis. Arthritis Rheum 2005; 52:856-64.

39. Hou J, Schindler U, Henzel WJ, Ho TC, Brasseur M, McKnight SL. An interleukin-4-induced transcription factor: IL-4 Stat. Science 1994; 265:1701-6.

40. Lin JX, Migone TS, Tsang M, Friedmann M, Weatherbee JA, Zhou L, et al. The role of shared receptor motifs and common Stat proteins in the generation of cytokine pleiotropy and redundancy by IL-2, IL-4, IL-7, IL-13, and IL-15. Immunity 1995; 2:331-9.

41. Ozaki K, Spolski R, Feng CG, Qi CF, Cheng J, Sher A, et al. A critical role for IL-21 in regulating immunoglobulin production. Science 2002; 298:1630-4.

42. Zeng R, Spolski R, Finkelstein SE, Oh S, Kovanen PE, Hinrichs CS, et al. Synergy of IL-21 and IL-15 in regulating CD8+ T cell expansion and function. J Exp Med 2005; 201:139-48.

43. Sivori S, Cantoni C, Parolini S, Marcenaro E, Conte R, Moretta L, et al. IL-21 induces both rapid maturation of human CD34+ cell precursors towards NK cells and acquisition of surface killer Ig-like receptors. Eur J Immunol 2003; 33:3439-47.

44. Brady J, Hayakawa Y, Smyth MJ, Nutt SL. IL-21 induces the functional maturation of murine NK cells. J Immunol 2004; 172:2048-58.

45. Pene J, Gauchat JF, Lecart S, Drouet E, Guglielmi P, Boulay V, et al. Cutting edge: IL-21 is a switch factor for the production of IgG1 and IgG3 by human B cells. J Immunol 2004; 172:5154-7.

46. Kuhn R, Rajewsky K, Muller W. Generation and analysis of interleukin-4 deficient mice. Science 1991; 254:707-10.

47. Suto A, Nakajima H, Hirose K, Suzuki K, Kagami S, Seto Y, et al. Interleukin 21 prevents antigen-induced IgE production by inhibiting germ line C(epsilon) transcription of IL-4-stimulated B cells. Blood 2002; 100:4565-73.

48. Kotlarz D, Zietara N, Uzel G, Weidemann T, Braun CJ, Diestelhorst J, et al. Loss-of-function mutations in the IL-21 receptor gene cause a primary immunodeficiency syndrome. J Exp Med 2013; 210:433-43.

49. Rodrigues F, Davies EG, Harrison P, McLauchlin J, Karani J, Portmann B, et al. Liver disease in children with primary immunodeficiencies. J Pediatr 2004; 145:333-9.

50. Elinav E, Strowig T, Kau AL, Henao-Mejia J, Thaiss CA, Booth CJ, et al. NLRP6 inflamma-some regulates colonic microbial ecology and risk for colitis. Cell 2011; 145:745-57.

51. Jostins L, Ripke S, Weersma RK, Duerr RH, McGovern DP, Hui KY, et al. Host-microbe interactions have shaped the genetic architecture of inflammatory bowel disease. Nature 2012; 491:119-24.

52. Rankin AL, MacLeod H, Keegan S, Andreyeva T, Lowe L, Bloom L, et al. IL-21 receptor is critical for the development of memory B cell responses. J Immunol 2011; 186:667-74.

53. Spolski R, Kim HP, Zhu W, Levy DE, Leonard WJ. IL-21 mediates suppressive effects via its induction of IL-10. J Immunol 2009; 182:2859-67.

54. Kotlarz D, Beier R, Murugan D, Diestelhorst J, Jensen O, Boztug K, et al. Loss of interleukin-10 signaling and infantile inflammatory bowel disease: implications for diagnosis and therapy. Gastroenterology 2012; 143:347-55.

55. Glocker EO, Frede N, Perro M, Sebire N, Elawad M, Shah N, et al. Infant colitis--it's in the genes. Lancet 2010; 376:1272.

56. Li J, Pan HF, Cen H, Tian J, Ma Y, Tao JH, et al. Interleukin-21 as a potential therapeutic target for systemic lupus erythematosus. Mol Biol Rep 2011; 38:4077-81.

57. Sarra M, Franze E, Pallone F, Monteleone G. Targeting interleukin-21 in inflammatory diseases. Expert Opin Ther Targets 2011; 15:695-702.

58. Yuan FL, Hu W, Lu WG, Li X, Li JP, Xu RS, et al. Targeting interleukin-21 in rheumatoid arthritis. Mol Biol Rep 2011; 38:1717-21.

59. Sivendran S, Glodny B, Pan M, Merad M, Saenger Y. Melanoma immunotherapy. Mt Sinai J Med 2010; 77:620-42.

60. Hashmi MH, Van Veldhuizen PJ. Interleukin-21: updated review of Phase I and II clinical trials in metastatic renal cell carcinoma, metastatic melanoma and relapsed/refractory indolent non-Hodgkin's lymphoma. Expert Opin Biol Ther 2010; 10:807-17.

61. Monteleone G, Pallone F, Macdonald TT. Interleukin-21 as a new therapeutic target for immune-mediated diseases. Trends Pharmacol Sci 2009; 30:441-7.

62. Schmidt H, Brown J, Mouritzen U, Selby P, Fode K, Svane IM, et al. Safety and clinical effect of subcutaneous human interleukin-21 in patients with metastatic melanoma or renal cell carcinoma: a phase I trial. Clin Cancer Res 2010; 16:5312-9.

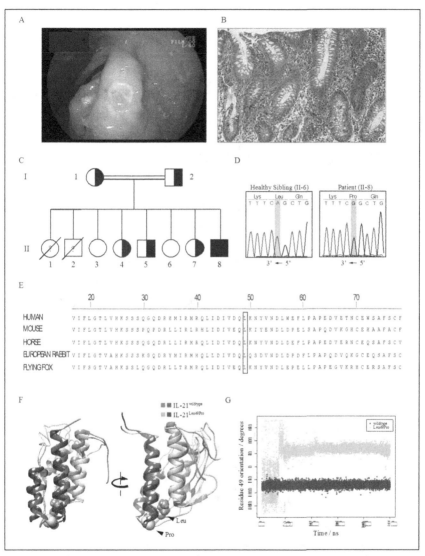

Figure 7:   Identification of IL21 deficiency. Colonoscopy (A). Histology consistent with Crohn's disease (B). Pedigree of index family; black filling marks IL21[Leu49Pro] segregation pattern (C). Sanger Chromatograms displaying the missense mutation in *IL21* in the patient (II-8) and a healthy sibling (II-6) (D). Amino acid sequence conservation of IL21[Leu49Pro] among different species (E). Structure of mutant IL21[Leu49Pro] overlapped with IL21[wildtype] (F). Orientation of the residue 49 in simulations of wildtype (brown) and IL21[Leu49Pro] (blue) (G).

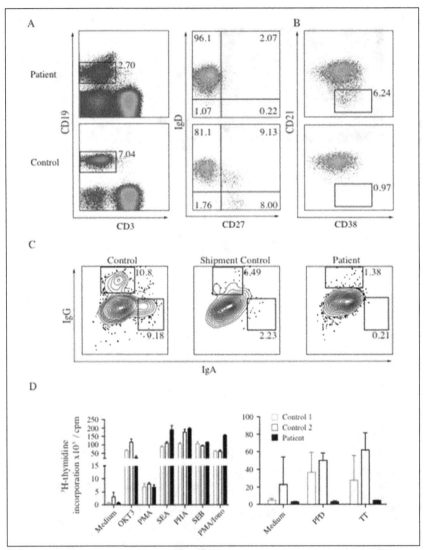

Figure 8: Immunological phenotype of the patient. Proportion of total B cells, and IgD⁺CD27⁺ and
IgD⁻CD27⁺ memory B cells in peripheral blood from the patient (A, upper panel), as well
as transitional B cells (B) compared to a healthy donor. Percentage of IgG⁺ and IgA⁺
class-switched cells in peripheral blood from patient and controls (C). T cell proliferation;
stimulation with for 3 (D, left panel) and 7 days (D, right panel).

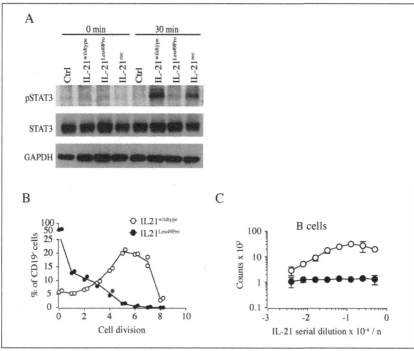

Figure 9: Functional consequences of IL21 deficiency. Western blot of pSTAT3 in Jurkat cells after stimulation with IL21^{wildtype}, IL21^{Leu49Pro}, and commercially available IL21 (IL21^{rec}) (A). FACS-based proliferation analysis of CFSE-labeled cord blood-derived CD19^{+} B cells after stimulation with IL21^{wildtype} (open circles) and IL21^{Leu49Pro} (closed circles) (B). IL21-dependent proliferation of cord blood-derived B cells 6 days after stimulation with IL21^{wildtype} (open circles) or IL21^{Leu49Pro} (closed circles) (C).

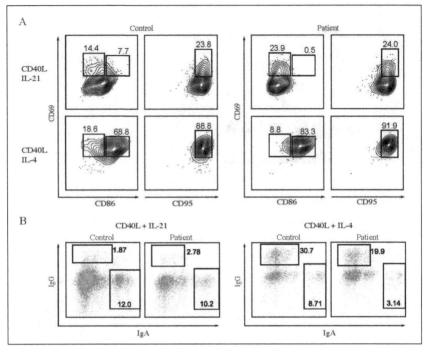

Figure 10: Normal activation and class switch recombination potential of IL21-deficient B cells. Flow cytometric analysis of control and patient PBMCs stimulated either with CD40L and IL21 (A, upper panel) or with CD40L and IL4 (A, lower panel). CD19⁺ B cells were stained for activation markers CD69, CD86 and CD95 after 3 day stimulation (A). Capacity of control and patient CD19⁺ B cells to undergo class switch recombination into IgG⁺ and IgA⁺ cells after 6 days of stimulation (B).

4 Discussion

4.1 Contribution to the field of primary immunodeficiencies

Primary immunodeficiencies are complex and diverse diseases. Although the incidence and prevalence of severe forms is not high, the identification of underlying genetic causes teaches us about non-redundant molecular mechanism of immune defense and host-pathogen interactions (Ochs & Hitzig, 2012).

Before the advancement of sequencing technologies, PIDs were only recognized in severe forms or as parts of characteristic syndromes (Milner & Holland, 2013). In the past years, the development of high throughput sequencing technologies enabled the discovery of PIDs with specific or subtle phenotypes, which often manifest during the first decade of life or during adolescence. Interestingly, many recently discovered PIDs do not have a corresponding animal model, reflecting the fact that the immune system is shaped in a constant intricate interplay with pathogens and environmental factors.

Here, we employed high-throughput sequencing technologies in combination with homozygosity mapping in a group of patients presenting with immunodeficiency, autoimmunity and / or lymphoproliferation and defective class-switch. We were able to identify two novel PIDs and increase the spectrum of patients with CD27 deficiency, for which before only a single family was published. Moreover, in the case of PKCδ and IL-21 deficiency we went on to discover the underlying mechanisms to explain the clinical picture of the disease.

We believe, that our work of the past four years has not only provided a molecular diagnosis for in total 10 patients, suffering from a previously unknown disease but has also helped to understand basic mechanisms of the immune system. Moreover, with the discovery of the underlying defect, therapy options have come into place, which had not been considered before, especially in the case of IL-21 deficiency. We hope, that follow-up studies will help to better characterize these diseases and to identify the best possible treatment option for these patients.

In the following chapters afore mentioned discoveries are described and discussed in more detail, referring to the basic biology background of the discovered diseases followed by discussing novel findings and placing them into context of prior knowledge from the literature.

4.2 Combined immunodeficiency with life threatening EBV-associated lymphoproliferative disorder in patients lacking functional CD27.

4.2.1 CD27 biology

CD27 is expressed on early thymocytes, naïve CD4 and CD8 cells (Nolte et al, 2009) and is commonly used as a marker for memory B cells (Klein et al, 1998). CD27 is a member of the TNF receptor (TNFR) superfamily and is known to interact with its unique ligand, CD70, a membrane-bound homotrimeric type II membrane protein (Lens et al, 1998). Binding of CD70 induces CD27 trimerization and thus initiation of intracellular signaling (Nolte et al, 2009). Moreover, it has been shown that upon binding of CD70, a truncated form of CD27 is released possibly cleaved by a membrane-linked protease (Loenen et al, 1992). Interestingly, increased levels of soluble CD27 have been found in patients with autoimmune diseases or viral infections (Lens et al, 1998).

On the other hand, CD27 activation induces intracellular signaling via TNFR-associated factor (TRAF) 2 and 5, which both get ubiquitinated after CD70 binding (Nolte et al, 2009). Consequently, both canonical and non-canonical NFκB pathways get activated (Ramakrishnan et al, 2004). However, it has been shown that the c-Jun terminal kinase (JNK)-signaling cascade (Akiba et al, 1998; Gravestein et al, 1998) as well as intracellular mediators of apoptosis (Prasad et al, 1997; Spinicelli et al, 2002) get activated upon CD70 binding (Nolte et al, 2009). In a mouse model it has been demonstrated that stimulation with an agonistic CD27 antibody induces proliferation and differentiation of T and B cells. Moreover, CD27 signaling seems to result in induction of TH1 differentiation in mice (Nolte et al, 2009).

4.2.2   CD27 deficiency in the context of other PIDs with lymphoproliferation

The first description of CD27 deficiency consisted of two brothers of a consanguineous Morrocan family who presented with EBV-associated immunodeficiency and lack of expression of CD27 on memory B cells. Capillary sequencing of *CD27* revealed a homozygous stopgain mutation (p.W8X) (van Montfrans et al, 2012). One patient presented with aplastic anemia and died of gram-positive sepsis. The other patient exhibited hypogamma-globulinemia with impaired specific antibody production. Both patients however showed lymphadenopathy, hepatosplenomegaly and lacked seroconversion for EBV-nuclear antigen (van Montfrans et al, 2012).

In our 8 patients described, the phenotype varied from asymptomatic borderline hypogammaglobulinemia to EBV-LPD, with progression to T and B cell lymphomas (Salzer et al, 2013a). These clinical features resemble other syndromes with increased susceptibility to EBV-LPD such as, among others, ITK deficiency (Huck et al, 2009), XIAP- (Rigaud et al, 2006) and SAP deficiency (Coffey et al, 1998). Interestingly, in all of these diseases including CD27 deficiency patients exhibit severely reduced to absent numbers of iNKT cells during active EBV-LPD (Ghosh et al, 2014). Therefore a critical role for iNKT cells has been suggested in controlling EBV infections (Chung et al, 2013). Recently our lab published a patient with ITK deficiency diagnosed prior to EBV infection and without LPD, who presented with CD4 lymphopenia and showed absence of iNKT cells, indicating the necessity of ITK for iNKT cell development (Serwas et al, 2014). Nevertheless, how and at which point during development CD27 influences iNKT cells remains to be clarified.

Interestingly, all 8 patients showed the exact same genetic mutation but presented high variability in the clinical presentation as well as spectrum of diseases. Clinical presentation of CD27 deficiency ranged from asymptomatic hypogammaglobulinemia to the development of both T and B cell malignancies (Salzer et al, 2013). As already discussed in the manuscript, it is hypothesized that "timing and tuning" of co-stimulatory signals in the course of the infection may be crucial to shape the immune response towards control or lympho-proliferation (Nolte et al, 2009). However, the precise mechanism by which CD27 facilitates EBV-LPD remains to be discovered.

4.3   B cell deficiency and severe autoimmunity caused by deficiency of protein kinase C δ.

4.3.1   PKCδ biology

The protein kinase C (PKC) family of serine/threonine kinases executes key roles in a plethora of cellular processes, including cell proliferation, apoptosis, and differentiation (Wu-Zhang et al, 2012). The PKC family can be divided in 3 subfamilies: conventional PKCs (cPKC), novel PKCs (nPKC) and atypical PKCs (aPKC) (Wu-Zhang et al, 2012).

PKCδ is a 78kDa protein with 676 amino acids, belongs to the novel PKC group and is a calcium-independent, phospholipid-dependent, serine/threonine kinase. The protein consists of a regulatory and a catalytic domain. PKCδ also contains five variable regions (V), where the variable region 3 (V3) acts as a hinge region between catalytic and regulatory domains. The C1 motif contains DAG (diacylglycerol)/PMA (Phorbol 12-myristate 13-acetate) binding sequences, which enable PKCδ binding to membranes (Cho, 2001). Although PKCδ has a C2-like region, this domain lacks the essential Ca^{2+} coordinating acidic residues that allow classical PKCs to bind Ca^{2+} (Pappa et al, 1998). C3 and C4 domains are needed for ATP/substrate binding and thus for the catalytic activity of the enzyme.

A pseudo substrate between C1 and C2 motifs retains PKCδ in an inactive conformation, thus blocking access to the substrate-binding pocket. When PKCδ is activated by proteolytic cleavage, a 40kDa fragment is generated which can translocate to mitochondria and/or nucleus (Cho, 2001; Hurley & Misra, 2000; Steinberg, 2004). Three specific sites need to be phosphorylated so that the kinase can be fully active: auto-phosphorylation at Ser643 (turn motif), Thr505 (activation loop of the kinase domain) and Ser662 (hydrophobic region)(Steinberg, 2004). Moreover, PKCδ can be phosphorylated by tyrosine kinases at eight Tyr residues. Tyr155 phosphorylation seems to be important for the inhibitory effect of PKCδ on cell proliferation (Sun et al, 2000; Szallasi et al, 1995). Tyrosine phosphorylation on the hinge and activation regions results in PKCδ activation and differential subcellular distribution onto membranes (Blake et al, 1999; Konishi et al, 1997). Conversely, phosphorylation of Tyr155 and Tyr187 promote the anti-apoptotic effect of PKCδ resulting in an increase in cell proliferation in response to PMA (Kronfeld et al, 2000).

4.3.2   PKCδ activation

PKCδ is activated downstream of a variety of stimuli including stress response to oxidative stress, DNA damage or ultra violet radiation (Zhao et al, 2012) (Figure 4). It is involved in signaling downstream of the BCR, interferon (IFN) receptors (Deb et al, 2003; Uddin et al, 2002) the insulin receptor (Braiman et al, 1999) and many others. PKCδ can be phosphorylated by various kinases leading to different phosphorylation patterns and possibly resulting in differential activation of downstream targets. After DAG binding, Ser/Thr phosphorylation by PDK1 and other upstream kinases including PKCζ and mTOR (mammalian target of rapamycin), but also auto-phosphorylation (Durgan et al, 2007) leads to full kinase activation. Tyr residues of PKCδ are phosphorylated by Src kinase family members (SRC, LYN, FYN, LCK), PYK2 or growth factor receptors, fine-tuning kinase activity and downstream effects (Kikkawa et al, 2002) (Basu & Pal, 2010).

Although PKCδ is a known regulator of pleiotropic functions, the true effect of absence of PKCδ in humans was only uncovered when we identified biallelic mutations in *PRKCD* as the molecular cause of a novel primary immunodeficiency disorder with severe, SLE-like systemic autoimmunity (Salzer et al, 2013).

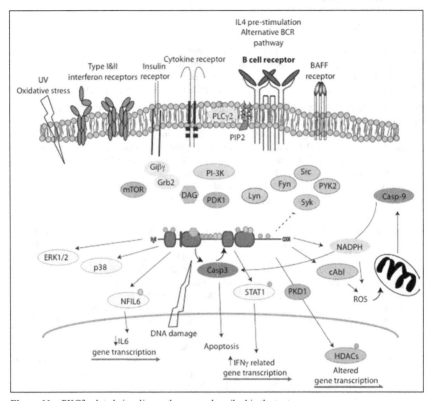

Figure 11: PKCδ related signaling pathways as described in the text.

4.3.3   Human PKCδ deficiency

Since our group initially described PKCδ deficiency in 2013 (Salzer et al, 2013), four additional patients from 2 unrelated kindreds have been published (Belot et al, 2013; Kuehn et al, 2013). All detected mutations were biallelic and led to loss of function or loss of expression of the corresponding protein product: c.1352+1G>A (splice-site),p.G510S and R614W.

Common features in all five patients include hepatosplenomegaly, lymphoproliferation and positive autoantibodies. Four patients also presented with lymphoproliferative features and/or kidney involvement. All patients developed symptoms before the age of 10 years. Recurrent infections were seen in 2 patients (Kuehn et al, 2013; Salzer et al, 2013). Immune phenotyping of peripheral blood leukocytes revealed mostly normal T cell numbers and function (Miyamoto et al, 2002). Circulating B cell counts were variable and reduced numbers of memory B cells were detected. Immunoglobulin levels varied as only 2 patients presented with elevated IgM levels. In peripheral lymphoid organs of two patients predominant B cell infiltration was observed. Treatment involved the use of corticosteroids and other immunosuppressants such as mycophenolate mofetil or rapamycin.

As specified above, all patients presented with systemic lupus erythematosus (SLE) or SLE-like autoimmunity and 4 out of 5 exhibited lymphoproliferative features and/or kidney involvement.

4.3.4   *PKCδ signaling and SLE*

Among others, PKCδ acts downstream of BTK and PLCγ2 (Guo et al, 2004). Recently, this pathway has been implicated in a novel PID with significant autoimmunity, displaying activating mutations in the *PLCγ2* gene, described by two independent groups in 2012 (Ombrello et al, 2012; Zhou et al, 2012). Moreover human PKCδ deficiency resembles the corresponding knock out mouse model, described in 2002 (Miyamoto et al, 2002). These mice showed lymphadenopathy, immune complex glomerulonephritis, splenomegaly and B cell infiltrations in several organs. Experimental studies revealed, as also demonstrated in PKCδ-deficient patients, increased production of IL-6, possibly leading to B cell hyper-proliferation.

SLE is a complex and to date still poorly understood disease and can be considered as the showcase for a systemic autoimmune mediated disease (Belot & Cimaz, 2012)).

In SLE, tolerance breakdown of both T and B cells can be observed (Wahren-Herlenius & Dorner, 2013). Already for some time it has been hypothesized that apoptosis defects may play an important role in the pathogenesis of SLE (Belot & Cimaz, 2012). In this model T and B cells are resistant to death signals, during central or peripheral tolerance induction (Belot & Cimaz, 2012)). Regarding T cells this hypothesis is evidenced by the fact that mutations in genes involved in the Fas pathway lead to ALPS or ALPS-like syndromes in humans (Oliveira et al, 2010). Interestingly, 4 out of 5 PKCδ deficient patients were clinically diagnosed with ALPS before the causative gene defect was discovered (Belot et al, 2013; Kuehn et al, 2013). For B cells, given the phenotype of Pkcδ knock out mice, a potential role for PKCδ in the pathogenesis of SLE was hypothesized. Given the multiple activities of PKCδ, it is not surprising that an altered PKCδ function contributes probably through several mechanisms to the immune dysregulation in SLE, although currently only few of them are sufficiently defined. Taken together the discovery of PKCδ deficient patients shed light on crucial functions of this kinase and define PKCδ as a critical regulator of immune homeostasis in man.

4.4   Early-onset inflammatory bowel disease and common variable immunodeficiency-like disease caused by IL-21 deficiency

4.4.1   *Discovery and biology of the IL-21/IL-21 receptor system*

The IL-21 receptor (IL-21R) was discovered by 2 groups in the year 2000 (Ozaki et al, 2000; Parrish-Novak et al, 2000), whereby they additionally identified the highly conserved WSXWS motive in the extracellular domain typically seen in type I cytokine receptors (Kotlarz et al, 2014). The IL-21 cytokine, on the other hand, is composed of four a-helices (A-

D), arranged in up-up-down-down constellation (Hamming et al, 2012). Due to the recent report of the crystal structure of the IL-21/IL-21R complex by Hamming et al. it is now known that the WSXWS motif as well as glycosylation of the IL-21R are critical for receptor binding and the interaction between IL-21 and the IL-21 receptor (IL-21R) takes place between amino-acids of helices A, C and a small part of the CD loop of IL-21 (Hamming et al, 2012). The IL-21R forms a heterodimeric complex with the common-γ chain, which is shared by IL-2, IL-4, IL-7, IL-9 and IL-15 (Rochman et al, 2009). Although the majority of binding energy is provided by the IL-21R, the interaction with the common-γ chain has been shown to be indispensable for signal transduction (Asao et al, 2001), evidenced by the fact that IL-21 mutants which cannot interact with the common-γ chain are agonists of IL-21 signaling (Kang et al, 2010).

IL-21 signals vial the Janus kinase (JAK)-signal transducer and activator of transcription (STAT) pathway (Rochman et al, 2009). IL-21 predominately activates STAT3 and 1, which distinguishes it from other cytokines of the common-γ chain-family but can phosphorylate STAT5A and B as well. Upon phosphorylation STATs dimerize and enter the nucleus to promote transcription of various target genes. Target genes of the phosphorylated STATs include, *Gzma, Gzmb, Il10, Socs1 and 3, Ifng, Cyclins a/b/e, Cxcr3 and 6, Bcl3, Jak3, Bim, Bcl6, Maf, Prdm1, Rorgt, Eomes, Il21,* and *Il21R* (Kotlarz et al, 2014). Thus IL-21 is critically involved in cell survival, cell-cycle regulation, cell migration, cellular activation, cytotoxicity and regulating its own expression (Kotlarz et al, 2014). Apart from the JAK-STAT pathway, IL-21 can also mediate activation of mitogen activated protein (MAP) kinase pathways or the Phosphoinositide (PI)-3 kinase pathway (Spolski & Leonard, 2014) via activation of JAK2 and 3.

The IL-21R is expressed on all hematopoietic cells, including epithelial cells, fibroblasts and keratinocytes. IL-21 is predominately produced by activated CD4 T cells (Kotlarz et al, 2014; Leonard & Spolski, 2005). Consistently, IL-21 exerts pleiotropic functions on almost all cells of the immune system (Spolski & Leonard, 2014). IL-21 is essential in the development of T_{FH} cells (Bauquet et al, 2009), T_{H17} cell differentiation (Linterman et al, 2010) and germinal center formation (Ozaki et al, 2004). Moreover, it is crucial for immunoglobulin class-switch and plasma cell differentiation of B cells (Ettinger et al, 2005). IL-21 is important for function and survival of CD8 T cells (Silver & Hunter, 2008) and has been shown to modulate NKT cell function (Coquet et al, 2007). Interestingly, IL-21 has been shown to be involved in the suppression of regulatory T cells by FOXP3 suppression (Li & Yee, 2008). More recently it became clear that IL-21 also plays important roles in the myeloid compartment by acting on macrophages (Vallieres & Girard, 2013), B-helper neutrophils (Puga et al, 2012) and dendritic cells (Wan et al, 2013).

4.4.2   Human IL-21R and IL-21 deficiency

In 2013, Kotlarz et al. (Kotlarz et al, 2014; Kotlarz et al, 2013) identified human IL-21R deficiency in two unrelated families with 4 affected individuals in total. The identified mutations in the *IL21R* gene were a missense mutation (c.G602T, p.Arg2201Leu) in patients 1 and 2 and a 6 base pair deletion (c.240_245delCTGCCA, p.Cys81_His82del) in patients 3 and 4.

Interestingly, all patients presented with severe liver disease due to chronic cholangitis caused by cryptosporidium infection (Kotlarz et al, 2014; Kotlarz et al, 2013). Two out of four patients were initially diagnosed with idiopathic liver fibrosis and listed for liver transplantation. Only in retrospect it became clear that these patients also suffered from a combined immunodeficiency mirrored by recurrent respiratory and gastrointestinal infections. Immunophenotyping of peripheral blood lymphocytes of these four patients showed normal T, B, and NK cell numbers (Kotlarz et al, 2014; Kotlarz et al, 2013). Detailed evaluation of B cells, however, revealed an increase of naïve B cells and a reduction of memory-switched B cells in three patients. All four patients also showed increased levels of IgE (Kotlarz et al, 2014; Kotlarz et al, 2013).

Experimental studies showed defective IL-21-induced STAT activation leading to defective IL-21 responses in lymphoid cells. Moreover, these patients also exhibited defective T cell proliferation towards specific antigens (Kotlarz et al, 2014; Kotlarz et al, 2013).

In a recent review by Kotlarz et al. (Kotlarz et al, 2014), three additional, to date still unpublished IL-21R deficient patients are mentioned. One patient presented with pulmonary tuberculosis, hepatosplenomegaly, chronic inflammatory skin disease and invasive fungal and viral infections as well as increased IgM levels and reduced class-switched CD19 cells. This patient died due to post HSCT complications. The detected mutation was a splice site conferring c.153-1G>T (Kotlarz et al, 2014). Another patient showed recurrent upper and lower respiratory tract infections and additionally presented with a B cell class switch defect. The patient was positive for *Pneumocystis jirovecii*, indicating a T cell deficiency. However, he did not show any cryptosporidium infection. This patient was transplanted at the age of 8 years. The detected mutation was a missense mutation (c.G602A, p.Arg201Gln). For the third patient no clinical description is available (Kotlarz et al, 2014).

In summary, the to date described IL-21R-deficient patients exhibit a T cell defect with reduced proliferation to specific antigens such as tetanus toxoid, but also a B cell defect, which is characterized by defective class switch and proliferation.

The up to now only case of IL-21 deficiency, described in the results section of this thesis on the other presented with early-onset inflammatory bowel disease and a CVID-like primary immunodeficiency. This patient also exhibited high IgE levels and a defective class switch in B cells, which was reversible *in vitro* after stimulation with wild type IL-21 (Salzer et al, 2014).

4.4.3 Concluding remarks

Interestingly, in contrast to other common γ-chain immunodeficiencies, IL21 or IL21R receptor deficiencies do not seem to be associated with a SCID phenotype. Still, all patients display a clear immunodeficiency with an increased susceptibility to infections and a higher mortality during childhood. Whereas IL-21R deficiency can be associated with severe liver disease due to cryptosporidium infection, the IL-21-deficient patient presented with inflammatory bowel disease but no cryptosporidium could be detected to date. Regarding the critical role of IL-21 in the modulation of immune homeostasis, early diagnosis and treatment is important and can be lifesaving.

In the case of IL-21R deficiency HSCT before cryptosporidium infection is crucial, as all patients transplanted with positive cryptosporidium suffered from severe transplant-related morbidities or died shortly after transplantation. For patients with IL-21 deficiency recombinant IL-21 represents an elegant alternative option, especially when the patient is not eligible for HSCT (see publication).

5 References

Ahonen P, Myllarniemi S, Sipila I, Perheentupa J (1990) Clinical variation of autoimmune polyendocrinopathy-candidiasis-ectodermal dystrophy (APECED) in a series of 68 patients. *N Engl J Med* **322**: 1829-1836

Aiuti A, Cattaneo F, Galimberti S, Benninghoff U, Cassani B, Callegaro L, Scaramuzza S, Andolfi G, Mirolo M, Brigida I, Tabucchi A, Carlucci F, Eibl M, Aker M, Slavin S, Al-Mousa H, Al Ghonaium A, Ferster A, Duppenthaler A, Notarangelo L, Wintergerst U, Buckley RH, Bregni M, Marktel S, Valsecchi MG, Rossi P, Ciceri F, Miniero R, Bordignon C, Roncarolo MG (2009) Gene therapy for immunodeficiency due to adenosine deaminase deficiency. *N Engl J Med* **360**: 447-458

Akashi K, Traver D, Miyamoto T, Weissman IL (2000) A clonogenic common myeloid progenitor that gives rise to all myeloid lineages. *Nature* **404**: 193-197

Akiba H, Nakano H, Nishinaka S, Shindo M, Kobata T, Atsuta M, Morimoto C, Ware CF, Malinin NL, Wallach D, Yagita H, Okumura K (1998) CD27, a member of the tumor necrosis factor receptor superfamily, activates NF-kappaB and stress-activated protein kinase/c-Jun N-terminal kinase via TRAF2, TRAF5, and NF-kappaB-inducing kinase. *The Journal of biological chemistry* **273**: 13353-13358

Al-Herz W, Bousfiha A, Casanova JL, Chapel H, Conley ME, Cunningham-Rundles C, Etzioni A, Fischer A, Franco JL, Geha RS, Hammarstrom L, Nonoyama S, Notarangelo LD, Ochs HD, Puck JM, Roifman CM, Seger R, Tang ML (2011) Primary immunodeficiency diseases: an update on the classification from the international union of immunological societies expert committee for primary immunodeficiency. *Front Immunol* **2**: 54

Al-Herz W, Bousfiha A, Casanova JL, Chatila T, Conley ME, Cunningham-Rundles C, Etzioni A, Franco JL, Gaspar HB, Holland SM, Klein C, Nonoyama S, Ochs HD, Oksenhendler E, Picard C, Puck JM, Sullivan K, Tang ML (2014) Primary immunodeficiency diseases: an update on the classification from the international union of immunological societies expert committee for primary immunodeficiency. *Front Immunol* **5**: 162

Aldrich RA, Steinberg AG, Campbell DC (1954) Pedigree demonstrating a sex-linked recessive condition characterized by draining ears, eczematoid dermatitis and bloody diarrhea. *Pediatrics* **13**: 133-139

Allen CD, Okada T, Cyster JG (2007) Germinal-center organization and cellular dynamics. *Immunity* **27**: 190-202

Allen RC, Armitage RJ, Conley ME, Rosenblatt H, Jenkins NA, Copeland NG, Bedell MA, Edelhoff S, Disteche CM, Simoneaux DK, et al. (1993) CD40 ligand gene defects responsible for X-linked hyper-IgM syndrome. *Science* **259**: 990-993

Anderson G, Moore NC, Owen JJ, Jenkinson EJ (1996) Cellular interactions in thymocyte development. *Annu Rev Immunol* **14**: 73-99

Antonarakis SE, Beckmann JS (2006) Mendelian disorders deserve more attention. *Nat Rev Genet* **7**: 277-282

Asao H, Okuyama C, Kumaki S, Ishii N, Tsuchiya S, Foster D, Sugamura K (2001) Cutting edge: the common gamma-chain is an indispensable subunit of the IL-21 receptor complex. *J Immunol* **167**: 1-5

Bamshad MJ, Ng SB, Bigham AW, Tabor HK, Emond MJ, Nickerson DA, Shendure J (2011) Exome sequencing as a tool for Mendelian disease gene discovery. *Nat Rev Genet* **12**: 745-755

Barrington RA, Pozdnyakova O, Zafari MR, Benjamin CD, Carroll MC (2002) B lymphocyte memory: role of stromal cell complement and FcgammaRIIB receptors. *J Exp Med* **196**: 1189-1199

Basu A, Pal D (2010) Two faces of protein kinase Cdelta: the contrasting roles of PKCdelta in cell survival and cell death. *TheScientificWorldJournal* **10:** 2272-2284

Bauquet AT, Jin H, Paterson AM, Mitsdoerffer M, Ho IC, Sharpe AH, Kuchroo VK (2009) The costimulatory molecule ICOS regulates the expression of c-Maf and IL-21 in the development of follicular T helper cells and TH-17 cells. *Nat Immunol* **10:** 167-175

Belot A, Cimaz R (2012) Monogenic forms of systemic lupus erythematosus: new insights into SLE pathogenesis. *Pediatric rheumatology online journal* **10:** 21

Belot A, Kasher PR, Trotter EW, Foray AP, Debaud AL, Rice GI, Szynkiewicz M, Zabot MT, Rouvet I, Bhaskar SS, Daly SB, Dickerson JE, Mayer J, O'Sullivan J, Juillard L, Urquhart JE, Fawdar S, Marusiak AA, Stephenson N, Waszkowycz B, M WB, Biesecker LG, G CMB, Rene C, Eliaou JF, Fabien N, Ranchin B, Cochat P, Gaffney PM, Rozenberg F, Lebon P, Malcus C, Crow YJ, Brognard J, Bonnefoy N (2013) Protein kinase cdelta deficiency causes mendelian systemic lupus erythematosus with B cell-defective apoptosis and hyperproliferation. *Arthritis and rheumatism* **65:** 2161-2171

Bidere N, Su HC, Lenardo MJ (2006) Genetic disorders of programmed cell death in the immune system. *Annu Rev Immunol* **24:** 321-352

Blake RA, Garcia-Paramio P, Parker PJ, Courtneidge SA (1999) Src promotes PKCdelta degradation. *Cell growth & differentiation : the molecular biology journal of the American Association for Cancer Research* **10:** 231-241

Bortin MM (1970) A compendium of reported human bone marrow transplants. *Transplantation* **9:** 571-587

Bousfiha AA, Jeddane L, Ailal F, Al Herz W, Conley ME, Cunningham-Rundles C, Etzioni A, Fischer A, Franco JL, Geha RS, Hammarstrom L, Nonoyama S, Ochs HD, Roifman CM, Seger R, Tang ML, Puck JM, Chapel H, Notarangelo LD, Casanova JL (2013) A phenotypic approach for IUIS PID classification and diagnosis: guidelines for clinicians at the bedside. *J Clin Immunol* **33:** 1078-1087

Boztug K, Schmidt M, Schwarzer A, Banerjee PP, Diez IA, Dewey RA, Bohm M, Nowrouzi A, Ball CR, Glimm H, Naundorf S, Kuhlcke K, Blasczyk R, Kondratenko I, Marodi L, Orange JS, von Kalle C, Klein C (2010) Stem-cell gene therapy for the Wiskott-Aldrich syndrome. *N Engl J Med* **363:** 1918-1927

Braiman L, Alt A, Kuroki T, Ohba M, Bak A, Tennenbaum T, Sampson SR (1999) Protein kinase Cdelta mediates insulin-induced glucose transport in primary cultures of rat skeletal muscle. *Molecular endocrinology* **13:** 2002-2012

Busslinger M (2004) Transcriptional control of early B cell development. *Annu Rev Immunol* **22:** 55-79

Canale VC, Smith CH (1967) Chronic lymphadenopathy simulating malignant lymphoma. *J Pediatr* **70:** 891-899

Carney JP, Maser RS, Olivares H, Davis EM, Le Beau M, Yates JR, 3rd, Hays L, Morgan WF, Petrini JH (1998) The hMre11/hRad50 protein complex and Nijmegen breakage syndrome: linkage of double-strand break repair to the cellular DNA damage response. *Cell* **93:** 477-486

Carvalho TL, Mota-Santos T, Cumano A, Demengeot J, Vieira P (2001) Arrested B lymphopoiesis and persistence of activated B cells in adult interleukin 7(-/)- mice. *J Exp Med* **194:** 1141-1150

Chen MR (2011) Epstein-barr virus, the immune system, and associated diseases. *Frontiers in microbiology* **2:** 5

Cheng MH, Anderson MS (2012) Monogenic autoimmunity. *Annu Rev Immunol* **30:** 393-427

Chi H (2012) Regulation and function of mTOR signalling in T cell fate decisions. *Nat Rev Immunol* **12:** 325-338

Cho W (2001) Membrane targeting by C1 and C2 domains. *The Journal of biological chemistry* **276:** 32407-32410

Chung BK, Tsai K, Allan LL, Zheng DJ, Nie JC, Biggs CM, Hasan MR, Kozak FK, van den Elzen P, Priatel JJ, Tan R (2013) Innate immune control of EBV-infected B cells by invariant natural killer T cells. *Blood* **122**: 2600-2608

Coffey AJ, Brooksbank RA, Brandau O, Oohashi T, Howell GR, Bye JM, Cahn AP, Durham J, Heath P, Wray P, Pavitt R, Wilkinson J, Leversha M, Huckle E, Shaw-Smith CJ, Dunham A, Rhodes S, Schuster V, Porta G, Yin L, Serafini P, Sylla B, Zollo M, Franco B, Bolino A, Seri M, Lanyi A, Davis JR, Webster D, Harris A, Lenoir G, de St Basile G, Jones A, Behloradsky BH, Achatz H, Murken J, Fassler R, Sumegi J, Romeo G, Vaudin M, Ross MT, Meindl A, Bentley DR (1998) Host response to EBV infection in X-linked lymphoproliferative disease results from mutations in an SH2-domain encoding gene. *Nat Genet* **20**: 129-135

Conley ME, Dobbs AK, Quintana AM, Bosompem A, Wang YD, Coustan-Smith E, Smith AM, Perez EE, Murray PJ (2012) Agammaglobulinemia and absent B lineage cells in a patient lacking the p85alpha subunit of PI3K. *J Exp Med* **209**: 463-470

Coquet JM, Kyparissoudis K, Pellicci DG, Besra G, Berzins SP, Smyth MJ, Godfrey DI (2007) IL-21 is produced by NKT cells and modulates NKT cell activation and cytokine production. *J Immunol* **178**: 2827-2834

Cunningham-Rundles C, Ponda PP (2005) Molecular defects in T- and B-cell primary immuno-deficiency diseases. *Nat Rev Immunol* **5**: 880-892

Cyster JG, Ansel KM, Reif K, Ekland EH, Hyman PL, Tang HL, Luther SA, Ngo VN (2000) Follicular stromal cells and lymphocyte homing to follicles. *Immunol Rev* **176**: 181-193

Deb DK, Sassano A, Lekmine F, Majchrzak B, Verma A, Kambhampati S, Uddin S, Rahman A, Fish EN, Platanias LC (2003) Activation of protein kinase C delta by IFN-gamma. *J Immunol* **171**: 267-273

Dent AL, Shaffer AL, Yu X, Allman D, Staudt LM (1997) Control of inflammation, cytokine expression, and germinal center formation by BCL-6. *Science* **276**: 589-592

Derbinski J, Gabler J, Brors B, Tierling S, Jonnakuty S, Hergenhahn M, Peltonen L, Walter J, Kyewski B (2005) Promiscuous gene expression in thymic epithelial cells is regulated at multiple levels. *J Exp Med* **202**: 33-45

Derbinski J, Schulte A, Kyewski B, Klein L (2001) Promiscuous gene expression in medullary thymic epithelial cells mirrors the peripheral self. *Nat Immunol* **2**: 1032-1039

Doria A, Zen M, Bettio S, Gatto M, Bassi N, Nalotto L, Ghirardello A, Iaccarino L, Punzi L (2012) Autoinflammation and autoimmunity: bridging the divide. *Autoimmun Rev* **12**: 22-30

Duraisingham SS, Buckland M, Dempster J, Lorenzo L, Grigoriadou S, Longhurst HJ (2014) Primary vs. secondary antibody deficiency: clinical features and infection outcomes of immunoglobulin replacement. *PloS one* **9**: e100324

Durandy A, Kracker S, Fischer A (2013) Primary antibody deficiencies. *Nat Rev Immunol* **13**: 519-533

Durgan J, Michael N, Totty N, Parker PJ (2007) Novel phosphorylation site markers of protein kinase C delta activation. *FEBS letters* **581**: 3377-3381

Engelhardt KR, McGhee S, Winkler S, Sassi A, Woellner C, Lopez-Herrera G, Chen A, Kim HS, Lloret MG, Schulze I, Ehl S, Thiel J, Pfeifer D, Veelken H, Niehues T, Siepermann K, Weinspach S, Reisli I, Keles S, Genel F, Kutukculer N, Camcioglu Y, Somer A, Karakoc-Aydiner E, Barlan I, Gennery A, Metin A, Degerliyurt A, Pietrogrande MC, Yeganeh M, Baz Z, Al-Tamemi S, Klein C, Puck JM, Holland SM, McCabe ER, Grimbacher B, Chatila TA (2009) Large deletions and point mutations involving the dedicator of cytokinesis 8 (DOCK8) in the autosomal-recessive form of hyper-IgE syndrome. *J Allergy Clin Immunol* **124**: 1289-1302 e1284

Ettinger R, Sims GP, Fairhurst AM, Robbins R, da Silva YS, Spolski R, Leonard WJ, Lipsky PE (2005) IL-21 induces differentiation of human naive and memory B cells into antibody-secreting plasma cells. *J Immunol* **175**: 7867-7879

Faitelson Y, Grunebaum E (2014) Hemophagocytic lymphohistiocytosis and primary immune deficiency disorders. *Clin Immunol* **155**: 118-125

Fazilleau N, Mark L, McHeyzer-Williams LJ, McHeyzer-Williams MG (2009) Follicular helper T cells: lineage and location. *Immunity* **30**: 324-335

Felgentreff K, Perez-Becker R, Speckmann C, Schwarz K, Kalwak K, Markelj G, Avcin T, Qasim W, Davies EG, Niehues T, Ehl S (2011) Clinical and immunological manifestations of patients with atypical severe combined immunodeficiency. *Clin Immunol* **141**: 73-82

Ferrari S, Giliani S, Insalaco A, Al-Ghonaium A, Soresina AR, Loubser M, Avanzini MA, Marconi M, Badolato R, Ugazio AG, Levy Y, Catalan N, Durandy A, Tbakhi A, Notarangelo LD, Plebani A (2001) Mutations of CD40 gene cause an autosomal recessive form of immunodeficiency with hyper IgM. *Proc Natl Acad Sci U S A* **98**: 12614-12619

Ferrari S, Zuntini R, Lougaris V, Soresina A, Sourkova V, Fiorini M, Martino S, Rossi P, Pietrogrande MC, Martire B, Spadaro G, Cardinale F, Cossu F, Pierani P, Quinti I, Rossi C, Plebani A (2007) Molecular analysis of the pre-BCR complex in a large cohort of patients affected by autosomal-recessive agammaglobulinemia. *Genes and immunity* **8**: 325-333

Filipovich A (2008) Hematopoietic cell transplantation for correction of primary immunodeficiencies. *Bone marrow transplantation* **42 Suppl 1**: S49-S52

Fischer A (2007) Human primary immunodeficiency diseases. *Immunity* **27**: 835-845

Fischer A, Le Deist F, Hacein-Bey-Abina S, Andre-Schmutz I, Basile Gde S, de Villartay JP, Cavazzana-Calvo M (2005) Severe combined immunodeficiency. A model disease for molecular immunology and therapy. *Immunol Rev* **203**: 98-109

Gardner JM, Fletcher AL, Anderson MS, Turley SJ (2009) AIRE in the thymus and beyond. *Curr Opin Immunol* **21**: 582-589

Gaspar HB, Aiuti A, Porta F, Candotti F, Hershfield MS, Notarangelo LD (2009) How I treat ADA deficiency. *Blood* **114**: 3524-3532

Gaspar HB, Cooray S, Gilmour KC, Parsley KL, Adams S, Howe SJ, Al Ghonaium A, Bayford J, Brown L, Davies EG, Kinnon C, Thrasher AJ (2011a) Long-term persistence of a polyclonal T cell repertoire after gene therapy for X-linked severe combined immunodeficiency. *Science translational medicine* **3**: 97ra79

Gaspar HB, Cooray S, Gilmour KC, Parsley KL, Zhang F, Adams S, Bjorkegren E, Bayford J, Brown L, Davies EG, Veys P, Fairbanks L, Bordon V, Petropoulou T, Kinnon C, Thrasher AJ (2011b) Hematopoietic stem cell gene therapy for adenosine deaminase-deficient severe combined immunodeficiency leads to long-term immunological recovery and metabolic correction. *Science translational medicine* **3**: 97ra80

Gatti RA, Meuwissen HJ, Allen HD, Hong R, Good RA (1968) Immunological reconstitution of sex-linked lymphopenic immunological deficiency. *Lancet* **2**: 1366-1369

Geha RS, Notarangelo LD, Casanova JL, Chapel H, Conley ME, Fischer A, Hammarstrom L, Nonoyama S, Ochs HD, Puck JM, Roifman C, Seger R, Wedgwood J (2007) Primary immunodeficiency diseases: an update from the International Union of Immunological Societies Primary Immunodeficiency Diseases Classification Committee. *J Allergy Clin Immunol* **120**: 776-794

Ghosh S, Bienemann K, Boztug K, Borkhardt A (2014) Interleukin-2-Inducible T-Cell Kinase (ITK) Deficiency - Clinical and Molecular Aspects. *J Clin Immunol* **34**: 892-899

Giblett ER, Anderson JE, Cohen F, Pollara B, Meuwissen HJ (1972) Adenosine-deaminase deficiency in two patients with severely impaired cellular immunity. *Lancet* **2**: 1067-1069

Glanzmann E, Riniker P (1950) [Essential lymphocytophthisis; new clinical aspect of infant pathology]. *Ann Paediatr* **175:** 1-32

Gravestein LA, Amsen D, Boes M, Calvo CR, Kruisbeek AM, Borst J (1998) The TNF receptor family member CD27 signals to Jun N-terminal kinase via Traf-2. *European journal of immunology* **28:** 2208-2216

Group of Pediatric I, Zelazko M, Liberatore D, Galicchio M, Perez N, Regairaz L, Oleastro M, Danielian S, Beroznik L, Di Giovani D, Riganti C, Diaz H, Cantisano C, Zorrilla LC, Nievas E (2013) Comment on: advances in primary immunodeficiency diseases in Latin America: epidemiology, research, and perspectives. Ann. N.Y. Acad. Sci. 1250: 62-72 (2012). *Annals of the New York Academy of Sciences* **1306:** 71-72

Guo B, Su TT, Rawlings DJ (2004) Protein kinase C family functions in B-cell activation. *Curr Opin Immunol* **16:** 367-373

Hamming OJ, Kang L, Svensson A, Karlsen JL, Rahbek-Nielsen H, Paludan SR, Hjorth SA, Bondensgaard K, Hartmann R (2012) Crystal structure of interleukin-21 receptor (IL-21R) bound to IL-21 reveals that sugar chain interacting with WSXWS motif is integral part of IL-21R. *The Journal of biological chemistry* **287:** 9454-9460

Hanna MG, Jr. (1964) An Autoradiographic Study of the Germinal Center in Spleen White Pulp during Early Intervals of the Immune Response. *Lab Invest* **13:** 95-104

Hardy RR, Carmack CE, Shinton SA, Kemp JD, Hayakawa K (1991) Resolution and characterization of pro-B and pre-pro-B cell stages in normal mouse bone marrow. *J Exp Med* **173:** 1213-1225

Haynes NM, Allen CD, Lesley R, Ansel KM, Killeen N, Cyster JG (2007) Role of CXCR5 and CCR7 in follicular Th cell positioning and appearance of a programmed cell death gene-1high germinal center-associated subpopulation. *J Immunol* **179:** 5099-5108

Hershfield MS (2003) Genotype is an important determinant of phenotype in adenosine deaminase deficiency. *Curr Opin Immunol* **15:** 571-577

Hogquist KA, Baldwin TA, Jameson SC (2005) Central tolerance: learning self-control in the thymus. *Nat Rev Immunol* **5:** 772-782

Hollander G, Gill J, Zuklys S, Iwanami N, Liu C, Takahama Y (2006) Cellular and molecular events during early thymus development. *Immunol Rev* **209:** 28-46

Huck K, Feyen O, Niehues T, Ruschendorf F, Hubner N, Laws HJ, Telieps T, Knapp S, Wacker HH, Meindl A, Jumaa H, Borkhardt A (2009) Girls homozygous for an IL-2-inducible T cell kinase mutation that leads to protein deficiency develop fatal EBV-associated lymphoproliferation. *J Clin Invest* **119:** 1350-1358

Hurley JH, Misra S (2000) Signaling and subcellular targeting by membrane-binding domains. *Annual review of biophysics and biomolecular structure* **29:** 49-79

Imai K, Slupphaug G, Lee WI, Revy P, Nonoyama S, Catalan N, Yel L, Forveille M, Kavli B, Krokan HE, Ochs HD, Fischer A, Durandy A (2003) Human uracil-DNA glycosylase deficiency associated with profoundly impaired immunoglobulin class-switch recombination. *Nat Immunol* **4:** 1023-1028

Jackson CE, Fischer RE, Hsu AP, Anderson SM, Choi Y, Wang J, Dale JK, Fleisher TA, Middelton LA, Sneller MC, Lenardo MJ, Straus SE, Puck JM (1999) Autoimmune lymphoproliferative syndrome with defective Fas: genotype influences penetrance. *Am J Hum Genet* **64:** 1002-1014

Janeway C (2008) Immunobiology.

Jordan MB, Allen CE, Weitzman S, Filipovich AH, McClain KL (2011) How I treat hemophagocytic lymphohistiocytosis. *Blood* **118:** 4041-4052

Kang HJ, Bartholomae CC, Paruzynski A, Arens A, Kim S, Yu SS, Hong Y, Joo CW, Yoon NK, Rhim JW, Kim JG, Von Kalle C, Schmidt M, Kim S, Ahn HS (2011) Retroviral gene therapy for X-linked chronic granulomatous disease: results from phase I/II trial. *Molecular therapy : the journal of the American Society of Gene Therapy* **19:** 2092-2101

Kang L, Bondensgaard K, Li T, Hartmann R, Hjorth SA (2010) Rational design of interleukin-21 antagonist through selective elimination of the gammac binding epitope. *The Journal of biological chemistry* **285:** 12223-12231

Kikkawa U, Matsuzaki H, Yamamoto T (2002) Protein kinase C delta (PKC delta): activation mechanisms and functions. *Journal of biochemistry* **132:** 831-839

Kildebeck E, Checketts J, Porteus M (2012) Gene therapy for primary immunodeficiencies. *Current opinion in pediatrics* **24:** 731-738

Klein U, Dalla-Favera R (2008) Germinal centres: role in B-cell physiology and malignancy. *Nat Rev Immunol* **8:** 22-33

Klein U, Rajewsky K, Kuppers R (1998) Human immunoglobulin (Ig)M+IgD+ peripheral blood B cells expressing the CD27 cell surface antigen carry somatically mutated variable region genes: CD27 as a general marker for somatically mutated (memory) B cells. *J Exp Med* **188:** 1679-1689

Kondo M, Weissman IL, Akashi K (1997) Identification of clonogenic common lymphoid progenitors in mouse bone marrow. *Cell* **91:** 661-672

Konishi H, Tanaka M, Takemura Y, Matsuzaki H, Ono Y, Kikkawa U, Nishizuka Y (1997) Activation of protein kinase C by tyrosine phosphorylation in response to H2O2. *Proceedings of the National Academy of Sciences of the United States of America* **94:** 11233-11237

Kopf M, Herren S, Wiles MV, Pepys MB, Kosco-Vilbois MH (1998) Interleukin 6 influences germinal center development and antibody production via a contribution of C3 complement component. *J Exp Med* **188:** 1895-1906

Kotlarz D, Zietara N, Milner JD, Klein C (2014) Human IL-21 and IL-21R deficiencies: two novel entities of primary immunodeficiency. *Current opinion in pediatrics* **26:** 704-712

Kotlarz D, Zietara N, Uzel G, Weidemann T, Braun CJ, Diestelhorst J, Krawitz PM, Robinson PN, Hecht J, Puchalka J, Gertz EM, Schaffer AA, Lawrence MG, Kardava L, Pfeifer D, Baumann U, Pfister ED, Hanson EP, Schambach A, Jacobs R, Kreipe H, Moir S, Milner JD, Schwille P, Mundlos S, Klein C (2013) Loss-of-function mutations in the IL-21 receptor gene cause a primary immunodeficiency syndrome. *J Exp Med* **210:** 433-443

Kronfeld I, Kazimirsky G, Lorenzo PS, Garfield SH, Blumberg PM, Brodie C (2000) Phosphorylation of protein kinase Cdelta on distinct tyrosine residues regulates specific cellular functions. *The Journal of biological chemistry* **275:** 35491-35498

Kuehn HS, Niemela JE, Rangel-Santos A, Zhang M, Pittaluga S, Stoddard JL, Hussey AA, Evbuomwan MO, Priel DA, Kuhns DB, Park CL, Fleisher TA, Uzel G, Oliveira JB (2013) Loss-of-function of the protein kinase C delta (PKCdelta) causes a B-cell lymphoproliferative syndrome in humans. *Blood* **121:** 3117-3125

Kuijpers TW, Bende RJ, Baars PA, Grummels A, Derks IA, Dolman KM, Beaumont T, Tedder TF, van Noesel CJ, Eldering E, van Lier RA (2010) CD20 deficiency in humans results in impaired T cell-independent antibody responses. *J Clin Invest* **120:** 214-222

Lederman HM (2000) The Clinical Presentation of Primary Immunodeficiency Diseases. *Clinical Focus on* **2**

Lens SM, Tesselaar K, van Oers MH, van Lier RA (1998) Control of lymphocyte function through CD27-CD70 interactions. *Seminars in immunology* **10:** 491-499

Leonard MF (1946) Chronic idiopathic hypoparathyroidism with superimposed Addison's disease in a child. *J Clin Endocrinol Metab* **6:** 493-506

Leonard WJ, Spolski R (2005) Interleukin-21: a modulator of lymphoid proliferation, apoptosis and differentiation. *Nat Rev Immunol* **5:** 688-698

Li FY, Chaigne-Delalande B, Kanellopoulou C, Davis JC, Matthews HF, Douek DC, Cohen JI, Uzel G, Su HC, Lenardo MJ (2011) Second messenger role for Mg2+ revealed by human T-cell immunodeficiency. *Nature* **475:** 471-476

Li Y, Yee C (2008) IL-21 mediated Foxp3 suppression leads to enhanced generation of antigen-specific CD8+ cytotoxic T lymphocytes. *Blood* **111:** 229-235

Li YS, Wasserman R, Hayakawa K, Hardy RR (1996) Identification of the earliest B lineage stage in mouse bone marrow. *Immunity* **5:** 527-535

Linterman MA, Beaton L, Yu D, Ramiscal RR, Srivastava M, Hogan JJ, Verma NK, Smyth MJ, Rigby RJ, Vinuesa CG (2010) IL-21 acts directly on B cells to regulate Bcl-6 expression and germinal center responses. *J Exp Med* **207:** 353-363

Liston A, Enders A, Siggs OM (2008) Unravelling the association of partial T-cell immunodeficiency and immune dysregulation. *Nat Rev Immunol* **8:** 545-558

Loenen WA, De Vries E, Gravestein LA, Hintzen RQ, Van Lier RA, Borst J (1992) The CD27 membrane receptor, a lymphocyte-specific member of the nerve growth factor receptor family, gives rise to a soluble form by protein processing that does not involve receptor endocytosis. *European journal of immunology* **22:** 447-455

MacLennan IC (1994) Germinal centers. *Annu Rev Immunol* **12:** 117-139

Mamanova L, Coffey AJ, Scott CE, Kozarewa I, Turner EH, Kumar A, Howard E, Shendure J, Turner DJ (2010) Target-enrichment strategies for next-generation sequencing. *Nat Methods* **7:** 111-118

Mandel TE, Phipps RP, Abbot AP, Tew JG (1981) Long-term antigen retention by dendritic cells in the popliteal lymph node of immunized mice. *Immunology* **43:** 353-362

Markert ML (1991) Purine nucleoside phosphorylase deficiency. *Immunodefic Rev* **3:** 45-81

McCusker C, Warrington R (2011) Primary immunodeficiency. *Allergy Asthma Clin Immunol* **7 Suppl 1:** S11

McKusick VA (2007) Mendelian Inheritance in Man and its online version, OMIM. *Am J Hum Genet* **80:** 588-604

Meffre E, Casellas R, Nussenzweig MC (2000) Antibody regulation of B cell development. *Nat Immunol* **1:** 379-385

Mendel G (1865) Versuche über Pflanzenhybriden. *Verhandlungen des naturforschenden Vereines in Brünn* **Bd. IV für das Jahr 1865:** 3–47

Miller JP, Izon D, DeMuth W, Gerstein R, Bhandoola A, Allman D (2002) The earliest step in B lineage differentiation from common lymphoid progenitors is critically dependent upon interleukin 7. *J Exp Med* **196:** 705-711

Milner JD, Holland SM (2013) The cup runneth over: lessons from the ever-expanding pool of primary immunodeficiency diseases. *Nat Rev Immunol* **13:** 635-648

Minegishi Y, Coustan-Smith E, Rapalus L, Ersoy F, Campana D, Conley ME (1999a) Mutations in Igalpha (CD79a) result in a complete block in B-cell development. *J Clin Invest* **104:** 1115-1121

Minegishi Y, Coustan-Smith E, Wang YH, Cooper MD, Campana D, Conley ME (1998) Mutations in the human lambda5/14.1 gene result in B cell deficiency and agammaglobulinemia. *J Exp Med* **187:** 71-77

Minegishi Y, Rohrer J, Coustan-Smith E, Lederman HM, Pappu R, Campana D, Chan AC, Conley ME (1999b) An essential role for BLNK in human B cell development. *Science* **286:** 1954-1957

Miyamoto A, Nakayama K, Imaki H, Hirose S, Jiang Y, Abe M, Tsukiyama T, Nagahama H, Ohno S, Hatakeyama S, Nakayama KI (2002) Increased proliferation of B cells and auto-immunity in mice lacking protein kinase Cdelta. *Nature* **416:** 865-869

Moraes-Vasconcelos D, Costa-Carvalho BT, Torgerson TR, Ochs HD (2008) Primary immune deficiency disorders presenting as autoimmune diseases: IPEX and APECED. *J Clin Immunol* **28 Suppl 1:** S11-19

Moshous D, Callebaut I, de Chasseval R, Corneo B, Cavazzana-Calvo M, Le Deist F, Tezcan I, Sanal O, Bertrand Y, Philippe N, Fischer A, de Villartay JP (2001) Artemis, a novel DNA double-strand break repair/V(D)J recombination protein, is mutated in human severe combined immune deficiency. *Cell* **105**: 177-186

Muller AM, Medvinsky A, Strouboulis J, Grosveld F, Dzierzak E (1994) Development of hematopoietic stem cell activity in the mouse embryo. *Immunity* **1**: 291-301

Myers LA, Patel DD, Puck JM, Buckley RH (2002) Hematopoietic stem cell transplantation for severe combined immunodeficiency in the neonatal period leads to superior thymic output and improved survival. *Blood* **99**: 872-878

Nehme NT, Pachlopnik Schmid J, Debeurme F, Andre-Schmutz I, Lim A, Nitschke P, Rieux-Laucat F, Lutz P, Picard C, Mahlaoui N, Fischer A, de Saint Basile G (2012) MST1 mutations in autosomal recessive primary immunodeficiency characterized by defective naive T-cell survival. *Blood* **119**: 3458-3468

Nieuwenhuis P, Opstelten D (1984) Functional anatomy of germinal centers. *Am J Anat* **170**: 421-435

Nishikawa Y, Hikida M, Magari M, Kanayama N, Mori M, Kitamura H, Kurosaki T, Ohmori H (2006) Establishment of lymphotoxin beta receptor signaling-dependent cell lines with follicular dendritic cell phenotypes from mouse lymph nodes. *J Immunol* **177**: 5204-5214

Nolte MA, van Olffen RW, van Gisbergen KP, van Lier RA (2009) Timing and tuning of CD27-CD70 interactions: the impact of signal strength in setting the balance between adaptive responses and immunopathology. *Immunol Rev* **229**: 216-231

Notarangelo LD (2009) Primary immunodeficiencies (PIDs) presenting with cytopenias. *Hematology Am Soc Hematol Educ Program*: 139-143

Notarangelo LD (2010) Primary immunodeficiencies. *J Allergy Clin Immunol* **125**: S182-194

O'Driscoll M, Cerosaletti KM, Girard PM, Dai Y, Stumm M, Kysela B, Hirsch B, Gennery A, Palmer SE, Seidel J, Gatti RA, Varon R, Oettinger MA, Neitzel H, Jeggo PA, Concannon P (2001) DNA ligase IV mutations identified in patients exhibiting developmental delay and immunodeficiency. *Mol Cell* **8**: 1175-1185

Ochs HD, Hitzig WH (2012) History of primary immunodeficiency diseases. *Current opinion in allergy and clinical immunology* **12**: 577-587

Oliveira JB, Bleesing JJ, Dianzani U, Fleisher TA, Jaffe ES, Lenardo MJ, Rieux-Laucat F, Siegel RM, Su HC, Teachey DT, Rao VK (2010) Revised diagnostic criteria and classification for the autoimmune lymphoproliferative syndrome (ALPS): report from the 2009 NIH International Workshop. *Blood* **116**: e35-40

Ombrello MJ, Remmers EF, Sun G, Freeman AF, Datta S, Torabi-Parizi P, Subramanian N, Bunney TD, Baxendale RW, Martins MS, Romberg N, Komarow H, Aksentijevich I, Kim HS, Ho J, Cruse G, Jung MY, Gilfillan AM, Metcalfe DD, Nelson C, O'Brien M, Wisch L, Stone K, Douek DC, Gandhi C, Wanderer AA, Lee H, Nelson SF, Shianna KV, Cirulli ET, Goldstein DB, Long EO, Moir S, Meffre E, Holland SM, Kastner DL, Katan M, Hoffman HM, Milner JD (2012) Cold urticaria, immunodeficiency, and autoimmunity related to PLCG2 deletions. *N Engl J Med* **366**: 330-338

Ozaki K, Kikly K, Michalovich D, Young PR, Leonard WJ (2000) Cloning of a type I cytokine receptor most related to the IL-2 receptor beta chain. *Proc Natl Acad Sci U S A* **97**: 11439-11444

Ozaki K, Spolski R, Ettinger R, Kim HP, Wang G, Qi CF, Hwu P, Shaffer DJ, Akilesh S, Roopenian DC, Morse HC, 3rd, Lipsky PE, Leonard WJ (2004) Regulation of B cell differentiation and plasma cell generation by IL-21, a novel inducer of Blimp-1 and Bcl-6. *J Immunol* **173**: 5361-5371

Palmer E (2003) Negative selection--clearing out the bad apples from the T-cell repertoire. *Nat Rev Immunol* **3**: 383-391

Pappa H, Murray-Rust J, Dekker LV, Parker PJ, Mcdonald NQ (1998) Crystal structure of the C2 domain from protein kinase C-delta. *Structure* **6**: 885-894

Parrish-Novak J, Dillon SR, Nelson A, Hammond A, Sprecher C, Gross JA, Johnston J, Madden K, Xu W, West J, Schrader S, Burkhead S, Heipel M, Brandt C, Kuijper JL, Kramer J, Conklin D, Presnell SR, Berry J, Shiota F, Bort S, Hambly K, Mudri S, Clegg C, Moore M, Grant FJ, Lofton-Day C, Gilbert T, Rayond F, Ching A, Yao L, Smith D, Webster P, Whitmore T, Maurer M, Kaushansky K, Holly RD, Foster D (2000) Interleukin 21 and its receptor are involved in NK cell expansion and regulation of lymphocyte function. *Nature* **408**: 57-63

Pieper K, Grimbacher B, Eibel H (2013) B-cell biology and development. *J Allergy Clin Immunol* **131**: 959-971

Porteus MH, Baltimore D (2003) Chimeric nucleases stimulate gene targeting in human cells. *Science* **300**: 763

Powell BR, Buist NR, Stenzel P (1982) An X-linked syndrome of diarrhea, polyendocrinopathy, and fatal infection in infancy. *J Pediatr* **100**: 731-737

Prasad KV, Ao Z, Yoon Y, Wu MX, Rizk M, Jacquot S, Schlossman SF (1997) CD27, a member of the tumor necrosis factor receptor family, induces apoptosis and binds to Siva, a proapoptotic protein. *Proc Natl Acad Sci U S A* **94**: 6346-6351

Puel A, Cypowyj S, Bustamante J, Wright JF, Liu L, Lim HK, Migaud M, Israel L, Chrabieh M, Audry M, Gumbleton M, Toulon A, Bodemer C, El-Baghdadi J, Whitters M, Paradis T, Brooks J, Collins M, Wolfman NM, Al-Muhsen S, Galicchio M, Abel L, Picard C, Casanova JL (2011) Chronic mucocutaneous candidiasis in humans with inborn errors of interleukin-17 immunity. *Science* **332**: 65-68

Puel A, Doffinger R, Natividad A, Chrabieh M, Barcenas-Morales G, Picard C, Cobat A, Ouachee-Chardin M, Toulon A, Bustamante J, Al-Muhsen S, Al-Owain M, Arkwright PD, Costigan C, McConnell V, Cant AJ, Abinun M, Polak M, Bougneres PF, Kumararatne D, Marodi L, Nahum A, Roifman C, Blanche S, Fischer A, Bodemer C, Abel L, Lilic D, Casanova JL (2010) Autoantibodies against IL-17A, IL-17F, and IL-22 in patients with chronic mucocutaneous candidiasis and autoimmune polyendocrine syndrome type I. *J Exp Med* **207**: 291-297

Puga I, Cols M, Barra CM, He B, Cassis L, Gentile M, Comerma L, Chorny A, Shan M, Xu W, Magri G, Knowles DM, Tam W, Chiu A, Bussel JB, Serrano S, Lorente JA, Bellosillo B, Lloreta J, Juanpere N, Alameda F, Baro T, de Heredia CD, Toran N, Catala A, Torrebadell M, Fortuny C, Cusi V, Carreras C, Diaz GA, Blander JM, Farber CM, Silvestri G, Cunningham-Rundles C, Calvillo M, Dufour C, Notarangelo LD, Lougaris V, Plebani A, Casanova JL, Ganal SC, Diefenbach A, Arostegui JI, Juan M, Yague J, Mahlaoui N, Donadieu J, Chen K, Cerutti A (2012) B cell-helper neutrophils stimulate the diversification and production of immunoglobulin in the marginal zone of the spleen. *Nat Immunol* **13**: 170-180

Radtke F, Wilson A, Stark G, Bauer M, van Meerwijk J, MacDonald HR, Aguet M (1999) Deficient T cell fate specification in mice with an induced inactivation of Notch1. *Immunity* **10**: 547-558

Ramakrishnan P, Wang W, Wallach D (2004) Receptor-specific signaling for both the alternative and the canonical NF-kappaB activation pathways by NF-kappaB-inducing kinase. *Immunity* **21**: 477-489

Randall KL, Lambe T, Johnson AL, Treanor B, Kucharska E, Domaschenz H, Whittle B, Tze LE, Enders A, Crockford TL, Bouriez-Jones T, Alston D, Cyster JG, Lenardo MJ, Mackay F, Deenick EK, Tangye SG, Chan TD, Camidge T, Brink R, Vinuesa CG, Batista FD, Cornall RJ, Goodnow CC (2009) Dock8 mutations cripple B cell immunological synapses, germinal centers and long-lived antibody production. *Nat Immunol* **10**: 1283-1291

Res P, Martinez-Caceres E, Cristina Jaleco A, Staal F, Noteboom E, Weijer K, Spits H (1996) CD34+CD38dim cells in the human thymus can differentiate into T, natural killer, and dendritic cells but are distinct from pluripotent stem cells. *Blood* **87**: 5196-5206

Revy P, Muto T, Levy Y, Geissmann F, Plebani A, Sanal O, Catalan N, Forveille M, Dufourcq-Labelouse R, Gennery A, Tezcan I, Ersoy F, Kayserili H, Ugazio AG, Brousse N, Muramatsu M, Notarangelo LD, Kinoshita K, Honjo T, Fischer A, Durandy A (2000) Activation-induced cytidine deaminase (AID) deficiency causes the autosomal recessive form of the Hyper-IgM syndrome (HIGM2). *Cell* **102**: 565-575

Rich KC, Arnold WJ, Palella T, Fox IH (1979) Cellular immune deficiency with autoimmune hemolytic anemia in purine nucleoside phosphorylase deficiency. *Am J Med* **67**: 172-176

Rigaud S, Fondaneche MC, Lambert N, Pasquier B, Mateo V, Soulas P, Galicier L, Le Deist F, Rieux-Laucat F, Revy P, Fischer A, de Saint Basile G, Latour S (2006) XIAP deficiency in humans causes an X-linked lymphoproliferative syndrome. *Nature* **444**: 110-114

Rochman Y, Spolski R, Leonard WJ (2009) New insights into the regulation of T cells by gamma(c) family cytokines. *Nat Rev Immunol* **9**: 480-490

Rothenberg EV (2000) Stepwise specification of lymphocyte developmental lineages. *Current opinion in genetics & development* **10**: 370-379

Rothenberg EV (2002) T-lineage specification and commitment: a gene regulation perspective. *Seminars in immunology* **14**: 431-440

Rothenberg EV, Telfer JC, Anderson MK (1999) Transcriptional regulation of lymphocyte lineage commitment. *BioEssays : news and reviews in molecular, cellular and developmental biology* **21**: 726-742

Salzer E, Daschkey S, Choo S, Gombert M, Santos-Valente E, Ginzel S, Schwendinger M, Haas OA, Fritsch G, Pickl WF, Forster-Waldl E, Borkhardt A, Boztug K, Bienemann K, Seidel MG (2013a) Combined immunodeficiency with life-threatening EBV-associated lympho-proliferative disorder in patients lacking functional CD27. *Haematologica* **98**: 473-478

Salzer E, Kansu A, Sic H, Majek P, Ikinciogullari A, Dogu FE, Prengemann NK, Santos-Valente E, Pickl WF, Bilic I, Ban SA, Kuloglu Z, Demir AM, Ensari A, Colinge J, Rizzi M, Eibel H, Boztug K (2014) Early-onset inflammatory bowel disease and common variable immunodeficiency-like disease caused by IL-21 deficiency. *J Allergy Clin Immunol* **133**: 1651-1659 e1612

Salzer E, Santos-Valente E, Klaver S, Ban SA, Emminger W, Prengemann NK, Garncarz W, Mullauer L, Kain R, Boztug H, Heitger A, Arbeiter K, Eitelberger F, Seidel MG, Holter W, Pollak A, Pickl WF, Forster-Waldl E, Boztug K (2013b) B-cell deficiency and severe autoimmunity caused by deficiency of protein kinase C delta. *Blood* **121**: 3112-3116

Salzer U, Bacchelli C, Buckridge S, Pan-Hammarstrom Q, Jennings S, Lougaris V, Bergbreiter A, Hagena T, Birmelin J, Plebani A, Webster AD, Peter HH, Suez D, Chapel H, McLean-Tooke A, Spickett GP, Anover-Sombke S, Ochs HD, Urschel S, Belohradsky BH, Ugrinovic S, Kumararatne DS, Lawrence TC, Holm AM, Franco JL, Schulze I, Schneider P, Gertz EM, Schaffer AA, Hammarstrom L, Thrasher AJ, Gaspar HB, Grimbacher B (2009) Relevance of biallelic versus monoallelic TNFRSF13B mutations in distinguishing disease-causing from risk-increasing TNFRSF13B variants in antibody deficiency syndromes. *Blood* **113**: 1967-1976

Savitsky K, Bar-Shira A, Gilad S, Rotman G, Ziv Y, Vanagaite L, Tagle DA, Smith S, Uziel T, Sfez S, Ashkenazi M, Pecker I, Frydman M, Harnik R, Patanjali SR, Simmons A, Clines GA, Sartiel A, Gatti RA, Chessa L, Sanal O, Lavin MF, Jaspers NG, Taylor AM, Arlett CF, Miki T, Weissman SM, Lovett M, Collins FS, Shiloh Y (1995) A single ataxia telangiectasia gene with a product similar to PI-3 kinase. *Science* **268**: 1749-1753

Schwarz K, Gauss GH, Ludwig L, Pannicke U, Li Z, Lindner D, Friedrich W, Seger RA, Hansen-Hagge TE, Desiderio S, Lieber MR, Bartram CR (1996) RAG mutations in human B cell-negative SCID. *Science* **274**: 97-99

Serwas NK, Cagdas D, Ban SA, Bienemann K, Salzer E, Tezcan I, Borkhardt A, Sanal O, Boztug K (2014) Identification of ITK deficiency as a novel genetic cause of idiopathic CD4+ T-cell lymphopenia. *Blood* **124**: 655-657

Shlomchik MJ, Weisel F (2012) Germinal center selection and the development of memory B and plasma cells. *Immunol Rev* **247**: 52-63

Silver JS, Hunter CA (2008) With a little help from their friends: interleukin-21, T cells, and B cells. *Immunity* **29**: 7-9

Sitnicka E, Bryder D, Theilgaard-Monch K, Buza-Vidas N, Adolfsson J, Jacobsen SE (2002) Key role of flt3 ligand in regulation of the common lymphoid progenitor but not in maintenance of the hematopoietic stem cell pool. *Immunity* **17**: 463-472

Sneller MC, Straus SE, Jaffe ES, Jaffe JS, Fleisher TA, Stetler-Stevenson M, Strober W (1992) A novel lymphoproliferative/autoimmune syndrome resembling murine lpr/gld disease. *J Clin Invest* **90**: 334-341

Spinicelli S, Nocentini G, Ronchetti S, Krausz LT, Bianchini R, Riccardi C (2002) GITR interacts with the pro-apoptotic protein Siva and induces apoptosis. *Cell death and differentiation* **9**: 1382-1384

Spolski R, Leonard WJ (2014) Interleukin-21: a double-edged sword with therapeutic potential. *Nature reviews Drug discovery* **13**: 379-395

Steinberg SF (2004) Distinctive activation mechanisms and functions for protein kinase Cdelta. *The Biochemical journal* **384**: 449-459

Stewart GS, Maser RS, Stankovic T, Bressan DA, Kaplan MI, Jaspers NG, Raams A, Byrd PJ, Petrini JH, Taylor AM (1999) The DNA double-strand break repair gene hMRE11 is mutated in individuals with an ataxia-telangiectasia-like disorder. *Cell* **99**: 577-587

Straus SE, Jaffe ES, Puck JM, Dale JK, Elkon KB, Rosen-Wolff A, Peters AM, Sneller MC, Hallahan CW, Wang J, Fischer RE, Jackson CM, Lin AY, Baumler C, Siegert E, Marx A, Vaishnaw AK, Grodzicky T, Fleisher TA, Lenardo MJ (2001) The development of lymphomas in families with autoimmune lymphoproliferative syndrome with germline Fas mutations and defective lymphocyte apoptosis. *Blood* **98**: 194-200

Sun X, Wu F, Datta R, Kharbanda S, Kufe D (2000) Interaction between protein kinase C delta and the c-Abl tyrosine kinase in the cellular response to oxidative stress. *The Journal of biological chemistry* **275**: 7470-7473

Szakal AK, Gieringer RL, Kosco MH, Tew JG (1985) Isolated follicular dendritic cells: cytochemical antigen localization, Nomarski, SEM, and TEM morphology. *J Immunol* **134**: 1349-1359

Szallasi Z, Denning MF, Chang EY, Rivera J, Yuspa SH, Lehel C, Olah Z, Anderson WB, Blumberg PM (1995) Development of a rapid approach to identification of tyrosine phosphorylation sites: application to PKC delta phosphorylated upon activation of the high affinity receptor for IgE in rat basophilic leukemia cells. *Biochemical and biophysical research communications* **214**: 888-894

Tang Q, Bluestone JA (2008) The Foxp3+ regulatory T cell: a jack of all trades, master of regulation. *Nat Immunol* **9**: 239-244

Tangye SG, Ma CS, Brink R, Deenick EK (2013) The good, the bad and the ugly - TFH cells in human health and disease. *Nat Rev Immunol* **13**: 412-426

Tarlinton D, Radbruch A, Hiepe F, Dorner T (2008) Plasma cell differentiation and survival. *Curr Opin Immunol* **20**: 162-169

Thiel J, Kimmig L, Salzer U, Grudzien M, Lebrecht D, Hagena T, Draeger R, Volxen N, Bergbreiter A, Jennings S, Gutenberger S, Aichem A, Illges H, Hannan JP, Kienzler AK, Rizzi M, Eibel H, Peter HH, Warnatz K, Grimbacher B, Rump JA, Schlesier M (2012) Genetic CD21 deficiency is associated with hypogammaglobulinemia. *J Allergy Clin Immunol* **129**: 801-810 e806

Uddin S, Sassano A, Deb DK, Verma A, Majchrzak B, Rahman A, Malik AB, Fish EN, Platanias LC (2002) Protein kinase C-delta (PKC-delta) is activated by type I interferons and mediates phosphorylation of Stat1 on serine 727. *The Journal of biological chemistry* **277**: 14408-14416

Vallieres F, Girard D (2013) IL-21 enhances phagocytosis in mononuclear phagocyte cells: identification of spleen tyrosine kinase as a novel molecular target of IL-21. *J Immunol* **190**: 2904-2912

van der Burg M, Gennery AR (2011) Educational paper. The expanding clinical and immunological spectrum of severe combined immunodeficiency. *Eur J Pediatr* **170**: 561-571

van Montfrans JM, Hoepelman AI, Otto S, van Gijn M, van de Corput L, de Weger RA, Monaco-Shawver L, Banerjee PP, Sanders EA, Jol-van der Zijde CM, Betts MR, Orange JS, Bloem AC, Tesselaar K (2012) CD27 deficiency is associated with combined immunodeficiency and persistent symptomatic EBV viremia. *J Allergy Clin Immunol* **129**: 787-793 e786

van Zelm MC, Reisli I, van der Burg M, Castano D, van Noesel CJ, van Tol MJ, Woellner C, Grimbacher B, Patino PJ, van Dongen JJ, Franco JL (2006) An antibody-deficiency syndrome due to mutations in the CD19 gene. *N Engl J Med* **354**: 1901-1912

van Zelm MC, Smet J, Adams B, Mascart F, Schandene L, Janssen F, Ferster A, Kuo CC, Levy S, van Dongen JJ, van der Burg M (2010) CD81 gene defect in humans disrupts CD19 complex formation and leads to antibody deficiency. *J Clin Invest* **120**: 1265-1274

Varon R, Vissinga C, Platzer M, Cerosaletti KM, Chrzanowska KH, Saar K, Beckmann G, Seemanova E, Cooper PR, Nowak NJ, Stumm M, Weemaes CM, Gatti RA, Wilson RK, Digweed M, Rosenthal A, Sperling K, Concannon P, Reis A (1998) Nibrin, a novel DNA double-strand break repair protein, is mutated in Nijmegen breakage syndrome. *Cell* **93**: 467-476

Vetrie D, Vorechovsky I, Sideras P, Holland J, Davies A, Flinter F, Hammarstrom L, Kinnon C, Levinsky R, Bobrow M, et al. (1993) The gene involved in X-linked agammaglobulinaemia is a member of the src family of protein-tyrosine kinases. *Nature* **361**: 226-233

Victora GD, Nussenzweig MC (2012) Germinal centers. *Annu Rev Immunol* **30**: 429-457

Victora GD, Schwickert TA, Fooksman DR, Kamphorst AO, Meyer-Hermann M, Dustin ML, Nussenzweig MC (2010) Germinal center dynamics revealed by multiphoton microscopy with a photoactivatable fluorescent reporter. *Cell* **143**: 592-605

Villa A, Santagata S, Bozzi F, Giliani S, Frattini A, Imberti L, Gatta LB, Ochs HD, Schwarz K, Notarangelo LD, Vezzoni P, Spanopoulou E (1998) Partial V(D)J recombination activity leads to Omenn syndrome. *Cell* **93**: 885-896

Vinuesa CG, Sanz I, Cook MC (2009) Dysregulation of germinal centres in autoimmune disease. *Nat Rev Immunol* **9**: 845-857

Wahren-Herlenius M, Dorner T (2013) Immunopathogenic mechanisms of systemic autoimmune disease. *Lancet* **382**: 819-831

Wan CK, Oh J, Li P, West EE, Wong EA, Andraski AB, Spolski R, Yu ZX, He J, Kelsall BL, Leonard WJ (2013) The cytokines IL-21 and GM-CSF have opposing regulatory roles in the apoptosis of conventional dendritic cells. *Immunity* **38**: 514-527

Waskow C, Paul S, Haller C, Gassmann M, Rodewald HR (2002) Viable c-Kit(W/W) mutants reveal pivotal role for c-kit in the maintenance of lymphopoiesis. *Immunity* **17**: 277-288

William J, Euler C, Christensen S, Shlomchik MJ (2002) Evolution of autoantibody responses via somatic hypermutation outside of germinal centers. *Science* **297**: 2066-2070

Wiskott A (1937) Familiärer, angeborener Morbus Werlhofii? *Monatsschrift für Kinderheilkunde*: 212-216

Wu Y, El Shikh ME, El Sayed RM, Best AM, Szakal AK, Tew JG (2009) IL-6 produced by immune complex-activated follicular dendritic cells promotes germinal center reactions, IgG responses and somatic hypermutation. *Int Immunol* **21**: 745-756

Wu-Zhang AX, Murphy AN, Bachman M, Newton AC (2012) Isozyme-specific interaction of protein kinase Cdelta with mitochondria dissected using live cell fluorescence imaging. *J Biol Chem* **287**: 37891-37906

Xing Y, Hogquist KA (2012) T-cell tolerance: central and peripheral. *Cold Spring Harbor perspectives in biology* **4**

Ye BH, Cattoretti G, Shen Q, Zhang J, Hawe N, de Waard R, Leung C, Nouri-Shirazi M, Orazi A, Chaganti RS, Rothman P, Stall AM, Pandolfi PP, Dalla-Favera R (1997) The BCL-6 proto-oncogene controls germinal-centre formation and Th2-type inflammation. *Nat Genet* **16:** 161-170

Yel L, Minegishi Y, Coustan-Smith E, Buckley RH, Trubel H, Pachman LM, Kitchingman GR, Campana D, Rohrer J, Conley ME (1996) Mutations in the mu heavy-chain gene in patients with agammaglobulinemia. *N Engl J Med* **335:** 1486-1493

Young LS, Rickinson AB (2004) Epstein-Barr virus: 40 years on. *Nat Rev Cancer* **4:** 757-768

Zhang Q, Davis JC, Lamborn IT, Freeman AF, Jing H, Favreau AJ, Matthews HF, Davis J, Turner ML, Uzel G, Holland SM, Su HC (2009) Combined immunodeficiency associated with DOCK8 mutations. *N Engl J Med* **361:** 2046-2055

Zhao M, Xia L, Chen GQ (2012) Protein kinase cdelta in apoptosis: a brief overview. *Archivum immunologiae et therapiae experimentalis* **60:** 361-372

Zheng Y, Josefowicz S, Chaudhry A, Peng XP, Forbush K, Rudensky AY (2010) Role of conserved non-coding DNA elements in the Foxp3 gene in regulatory T-cell fate. *Nature* **463:** 808-812

Zhou Q, Lee GS, Brady J, Datta S, Katan M, Sheikh A, Martins MS, Bunney TD, Santich BH, Moir S, Kuhns DB, Long Priel DA, Ombrello A, Stone D, Ombrello MJ, Khan J, Milner JD, Kastner DL, Aksentijevich I (2012) A hypermorphic missense mutation in PLCG2, encoding phospholipase Cgamma2, causes a dominantly inherited autoinflammatory disease with immunodeficiency. *Am J Hum Genet* **91:** 713-720

Zhou X, Bailey-Bucktrout SL, Jeker LT, Penaranda C, Martinez-Llordella M, Ashby M, Nakayama M, Rosenthal W, Bluestone JA (2009) Instability of the transcription factor Foxp3 leads to the generation of pathogenic memory T cells in vivo. *Nat Immunol* **10:** 1000-1007

6 Publications

Salzer E, Cagdas D, Hons M, Mace EM, Garncarz W, Petronczki ÖY, Platzer R, Pfajfer L, Bilic I, Ban SA, Willmann KL, Mukherjee M, Supper V, Hsu HT, Banerjee PP, Sinha P, McClanahan F, Zlabinger GJ, Pickl WF, Gribben JG, Stockinger H, Bennett KL, Huppa JB, Dupré L, Sanal Ö, Jäger U, Sixt M, Tezcan I, Orange JS, Boztug K. **RASGRP1 deficiency causes immunodeficiency with impaired cytoskeletal dynamics.**

Nat Immunol. 2016 Dec

Erman B, Bilic I, Hirschmugl T, **Salzer E**, Çağdaş DA, Esenboga S, Akcoren Z, Sanal O, Tezcan I, Boztug K. **Combined immunodeficiency with CD4 lymphopenia and sclerosing cholangitis caused by a novel loss-of-function mutation affecting IL21R.**

Haematologica. 2015 Mar 13

Woutsas S, Aytekin C, **Salzer E**, Conde CD, Apaydin S, Pichler H, Memaran-Dadgar N, Hosnut FO, Förster-Waldl E, Matthes S, Huber WD, Lion T, Holter W, Bilic I, Boztug K. **Hypomorphic mutation in TTC7A causes combined immunodeficiency with mild structural intestinal defects.**

Blood. 2015 Mar 5

Willmann KL, Klaver S, Doğu F, Santos-Valente E, Garncarz W, Bilic I, Mace E, **Salzer E**, Conde CD, Sic H, Májek P, Banerjee PP, Vladimer GI, Haskoloğlu S, Bolkent MG, Küpesiz A, Condino-Neto A, Colinge J, Superti-Furga G, Pickl WF, van Zelm MC, Eibel H, Orange JS, Ikincioğulları A, Boztuğ K. **Biallelic loss-of-function mutation in NIK causes a primary immunodeficiency with multifaceted aberrant lymphoid immunity.**

Nat Commun. 2014 Nov

Ban SA, **Salzer E**, Eibl MM, Linder A, Geier CB, Santos-Valente E, Garncarz W, Lion T, Ott R, Seelbach C, Boztug K, Wolf HM. **Combined immunodeficiency evolving into predominant CD4+ lymphopenia caused by somatic chimerism in JAK3.**

J Clin Immunol. 2014 Nov

Boztug K, Järvinen P, **Salzer E**, Racek T, Mönch S, Garncarz W, Gertz ME, Schäffer AE, Antonopoulos A, Haslam SM, Ziesenitz L, Puchałka J, Diestelhorst D, Appaswamy G, Lescoeur B, Giambruno R, Bigenzahn JW, Elling U, Pfeifer D, Domínguez Conde C, Albert M, Welte K, Brandes G, Sherkat R, van der Werff ten Bosch J, Rezaei N, Etzioni A, Bellanné-Chantelot C, Superti-Furga G, Penninger JM, Bennett KL, von Blume J, Dell A, Donadieu J, Klein C **JAGN1 deficiency causes aberrant myeloid cell homeostasis and congenital neutropenia**

Nat Genet. 2014 Sep

Salzer E, Kansu A, Sic H, Májek P, Ikincioğullari A, Dogu FE, Prengemann NK, Santos-Valente E, Pickl WF, Bilic I, Ban SA, Kuloğlu Z, Demir AM, Ensari A, Colinge J, Rizzi M, Eibl H, Boztug K. **Early-onset inflammatory bowel disease and common variable immunodeficiency-like disease caused by loss-of-function mutation in *IL21***

J Allergy Clin Immunol. 2014 Apr 17

Salzer E*, Santos-Valente E*, Klaver S, Ban SA, Emminger W, Prengemann NK, Garncarz W, Müllauer L, Kain R, Boztug H, Heitger A, Arbeiter K, Eitelberger F, Seidel MG, Holter W, Pollak A, Pickl WF, Förster-Waldl E#, Boztug K#.**B-cell deficiency and severe autoimmunity caused by deficiency of protein kinase Cδ.**

Blood. 2013 Apr 18 (* and # equal contribution)

Salzer E*, Daschkey S*, Choo S, Gombert M, Santos-Valente E, Ginzel S, Schwendinger M, Haas OA, Fritsch G, Pickl WF, Förster-Waldl E, Borkhardt A#, Boztug K#, Bienemann K, Seidel MG#. **Combined immunodeficiency with life-threatening EBV-associated lymphoproliferative disorder in patients lacking functional CD27.**

Haematologica. 2013 Mar 13 (* and # equal contribution)

Kratochwill K, Boehm M, Herzog R, Lichtenauer AM, **Salzer E**, Lechner M, Kuster L, Bergmeister K, Rizzi A, Mayer B, Aufricht C.

Alanyl-glutamine dipeptide restores the cytoprotective stress proteome of mesothelial cells exposed to peritoneal dialysis fluid;

Nephrol Dial Transplant. 2012 Mar 27

Riesenhuber A., Vargha R., Kratochwill K., Kasper D.C., **Salzer E.**; Aufricht C.

Peritoneal Dialysis Fluid induces p38 dependent Inflammation in Human mesothelial cells;

Peritoneal Dialysis International. 2011 May 31

Printed in the United States
By Bookmasters